T0200148

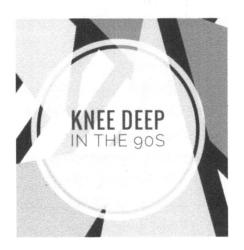

KNEE DEEP
IN THE 90S

Stop scrolling, start chilling:

Your Knee Deep in the 90s playlist.

The 90s

Activity Book

Chilled-out quizzes,
puzzles, colouring
and more …

@kneedeepinthe90s

POP PRESS

Welcome to a wonderful world of 1990s nostalgia and escapism!

In a time before social media and, dare I say it (because it makes me feel incredibly old), the internet, we were all living what we truly believed to be unique childhoods. In reality, we children of the nineties were, in fact, all living *identical* childhoods but completely oblivious to it – and oh, how happy we were in that state of oblivion!

Children born in the 1980s who grew up in the 1990s *are the last generation to know what life is like both with and without the internet.* Reminiscing about the nineties is far more than just nostalgia – it is a yearning for a pre-internet world before a technological revolution that changed our lives forever.

The 1990s were a very different world from the one in which we live today: not much opportunity for communication, apart from the landline, and much less in the way of entertainment – no YouTube or Netflix; nothing 'on demand' – we watched what was on a small number of TV channels at the time it was on or battled with a video recorder. A lot of the time, we had to create our own fun. We would listen patiently for *that* song to play on the radio so we could record it, only for the tape to get stuck or cut out mid-way through. We knew the feeling of disappointment when a toy was sold out forever.

We were, in many ways, the last of a disconnected generation and perhaps this is one of the reasons why feelings of 1990s nostalgia are ever growing. We're all seeking to achieve a bit of calm and time in a constantly connected world, to reminisce about an era that, looking back now, seems simpler in so many ways, and less flooded with endless, dizzying choice.

In 2022, I started an Instagram account called @kneedeepinthe90s. The response was amazing! It is now a real community of adults looking to celebrate all the things we loved as children and young people, and disconnect from everyday stress.

I receive messages all the time from people who follow the account telling me how much they enjoy taking a step back from their daily lives and responsibilities to reflect on a much simpler time – the Instagram feed has become a happy place for people to escape to. The good feelings that can be evoked from a simple childhood memory – such as a loved Christmas toy, the theme tune to a TV show you watched with your parents or the smell of a lip balm you remember buying on your first ever shopping trip with your friends – are what I want to share online, and also in this book.

So put away your phone, step away from the screens and enjoy the simple things for a few minutes. This is a 100 per cent analogue-age timeout.

I hope every page is a happy blast from your past. Find iconic toys, treats, music, moments, iconic TV, movies and people to colour, search for in word puzzles and remember in pop quizzes.

Victoria

@kneedeepinthe90s

P.S. Don't google the answers (pretend you're in the 90s and use your brain!).

COLOUR TIME

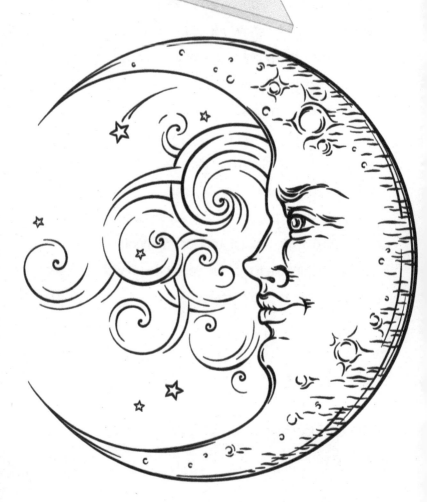

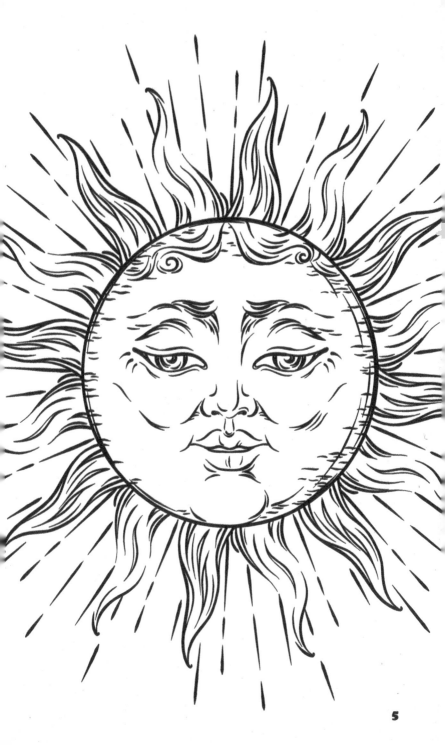

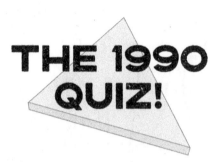

THE 1990 QUIZ!

1 Dannii Minogue played fictional character Emma Jackson in Australian TV series *Home and Away* but left in 1990 to launch her music career. Can you name her first single?

2 US book and TV series *Sweet Valley Twins* and *Sweet Valley High* followed the story of identical twins Jessica and Elizabeth Wakefield, but how many minutes apart were the twins born?

3 Name the song and artist most recognised for its use in the theme of *Baywatch*?

4 Australian TV series *Pugwall* followed the trials and tribulations of Peter Unwin George Wall and those of his band as they attempted to secure a record deal. What was the name of the band?

5 1990 saw the arrival of the British TV show *One Foot in the Grave*. Which character created the phrase 'I don't believe it!'?

6 In *Captain Planet and the Planeteers*, each Planeteer possesses a power related to the elements: wind, earth, water, fire – and what else?

7 Which Australian children's television series follows the adventures of a family who left their old life to live in a lighthouse in the fictional town of Port Niranda?

8 'World in Motion…' was sung by British group New Order with the members of the English national football team to celebrate their 1990 FIFA World Cup campaign. It famously features a guest rap by which ex-footballer?

9 1990 saw the reinvention of Kylie Minogue with a consciously more 'sexy' look, moving away from the girl-next-door persona that had come with her portrayal of Charlene on *Neighbours*. What was the breakout song from her *Rhythm of Love* album that came out that year?

10 Which cartoon began as a short segment on the *Tracy Ullman Show* and then started airing regularly as a programme on its own?

Answers on page 116

THE THINGS WE WORE

Baguette bag
Bucket hat
Butterfly clips
Cargo pants
Choker
Crop top
Double denim

Dr Martens
Dummy necklace
Jelly shoes
Mood ring
Pedal pushers
Platform shoes
Scrunchy

Slip dress
Snap band
Temporary tattoo
Thong
Wedges

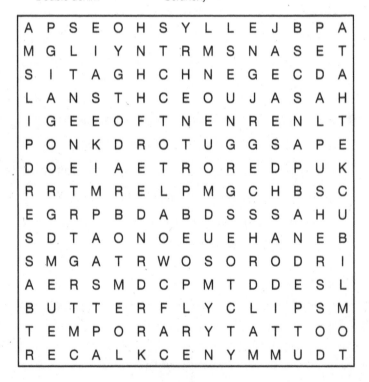

A	P	S	E	O	H	S	Y	L	L	E	J	B	P	A
M	G	L	I	Y	N	T	R	M	S	N	A	S	E	T
S	I	T	A	G	H	C	H	N	E	G	E	C	D	A
L	A	N	S	T	H	C	E	O	U	J	A	S	A	H
I	G	E	E	O	F	T	N	E	N	R	E	N	L	T
P	O	N	K	D	R	O	T	U	G	G	S	A	P	E
D	O	E	I	A	E	T	R	O	R	E	D	P	U	K
R	R	T	M	R	E	L	P	M	G	C	H	B	S	C
E	G	R	P	B	D	A	B	D	S	S	S	A	H	U
S	D	T	A	O	N	O	E	U	E	H	A	N	E	B
S	M	G	A	T	R	W	O	S	O	R	O	D	R	I
A	E	R	S	M	D	C	P	M	T	D	D	E	S	L
B	U	T	T	E	R	F	L	Y	C	L	I	P	S	M
T	E	M	P	O	R	A	R	Y	T	A	T	T	O	O
R	E	C	A	L	K	C	E	N	Y	M	M	U	D	T

Solution on page 121

Who is this icon of 1990s girl power?

Draw straight lines to join the stars and dots in numerical order. Each time you reach a hollow star, lift your pen and continue drawing from the next solid star.

Solution on page 137

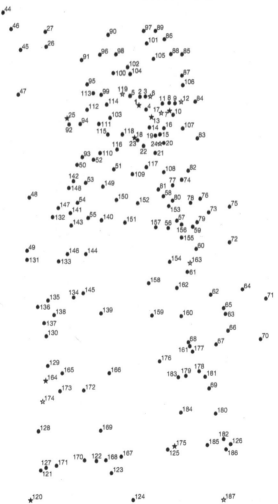

CROSSWORD 1

Solve the clues and discover the
1990s anagram in the shaded boxes!

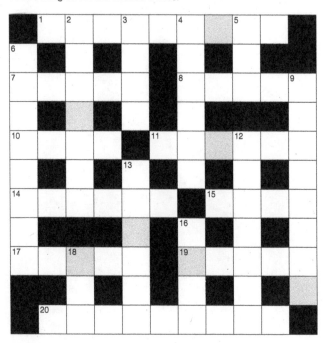

Across
1 Principal church (9)
7 Opts (5)
8 Will (5)
10 Maple or spruce, eg (4)
11 Feel pain (6)
14 Plan; mean (6)
15 Strong desire (4)
17 Fit a pane (5)
19 All-night parties (5)
20 Relating to the whole Earth (9)

Down
2 Extremely old (7)
3 Mess (4)
4 Athletic throwing event (6)
5 'I've got it!' (3)
6 Spluttering (8)
9 Generosity (8)
12 Eternally (7)
13 Unobserved (6)
16 Young troublemaker (4)
18 It's used for boring small holes (3)

Solution on page 131

COLOUR TIME

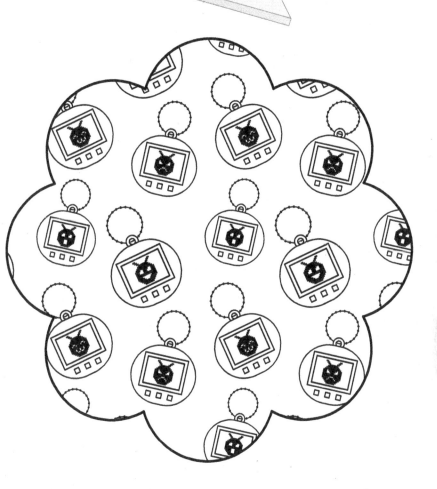

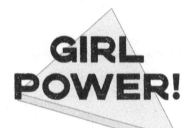

GIRL POWER!

Baby	Girl power	Sporty
Become one	Goodbye	Wannabe
Forever	Love	Zigazigah
Friendship	Posh	
Ginger	Scary	

```
O  I  M  F  O  R  N  E  W  E  I  R  I  O  T
C  I  E  O  R  Y  E  N  F  P  N  M  I  N  S
R  I  B  R  E  Y  E  O  I  O  A  R  G  P  H
E  O  A  E  W  O  O  E  E  S  A  G  O  A  Y
G  F  N  V  O  E  O  M  N  H  I  R  G  I  Y
I  G  N  E  P  A  O  O  S  N  T  I  I  B  B
G  V  A  R  L  G  E  C  G  Y  Z  S  E  O  A
A  O  W  W  R  R  O  E  H  A  F  R  A  F  B
B  A  R  F  I  Y  R  B  G  G  F  L  B  I  O
A  O  A  S  G  R  B  I  S  O  P  F  O  R  N
P  N  E  N  O  A  Z  Y  H  E  E  R  I  V  A
R  C  O  E  Y  C  B  E  O  E  R  L  S  A  E
I  D  R  S  O  S  O  F  O  I  Y  B  P  R  A
R  E  F  R  I  E  N  D  S  H  I  P  E  I  I
R  E  Y  R  A  O  O  G  O  O  D  B  Y  E  R
```

Solution on page 121

CROSSWORD 2

Solve the clues and discover the
1990s anagram in the shaded boxes!

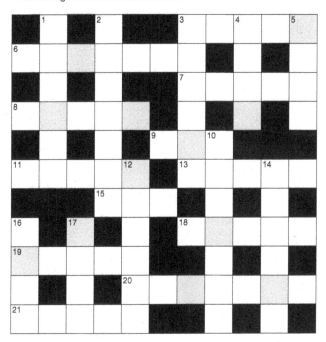

Across
- **3** Quality beef cut (5)
- **6** *Donkey Kong* villain (7)
- **7** Self-replicating computer program (5)
- **8** Flows like treacle (5)
- **9** Place to spend the night (3)
- **11** Bottom half of a semicolon (5)
- **13** Fault (5)
- **15** Bother (3)
- **18** Halt; ___ and desist (5)
- **19** Performing (5)
- **20** Enthusiastic (7)
- **21** States firmly (5)

Down
- **1** Late baroque style of decoration (6)
- **2** Quandary (7)
- **3** Reduction (6)
- **4** Messes up (4)
- **5** Touch with the lips (4)
- **10** Consisting of numbers (7)
- **12** Maxims (6)
- **14** Made it to the end (6)
- **16** Brainwave (4)
- **17** Chianti or Chablis (4)

Solution on page 131

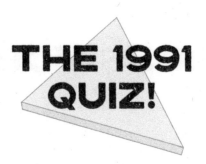

THE 1991 QUIZ!

1 What was the Spanish phrase made famous by the year's highest-grossing movie?

2 What was the full name of the character played by Melissa Joan Hart between 1991 and 1994 who explained it all?

3 In *Home Improvement*, what was the of the neighbour Tim Taylor talked to over the fence but we only ever saw his hat?

4 What are REM losing in their 1991 single?

5 Which Disney film became the first animated movie to be nominated for an Academy award?

6 MC Hammer made the Hammer dance famous in which song in 1991?

7 What song dominated the charts in the summer of 1991, going on to be one of the bestselling singles of all time?

8 What was the name of the platform game that kept us fixated on the progress of a spiny mammal that could run at rapid speed?

9 Which sitcom premiered and became quickly recognised for the catchphrases 'I'm the baby, gotta love me' and 'Not the mama!'?

10 Which era-defining soap aired its final episode after 14 seasons and a total of 357 shows?

Answers on page 116

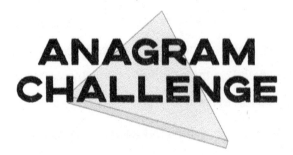

ANAGRAM CHALLENGE

Romcoms

Rearrange the letters below to reveal the title
of an iconic 90s romcom on each line.

1 LESS ELITE TENSE PALS (9, 2, 7)

◯◯◯◯◯◯◯◯◯
◯◯ ◯◯◯◯◯◯◯

2 I'M A GUY TO LOVE (5, 3, 4)

◯◯◯◯◯ ◯◯◯◯
◯◯◯◯

3 USE CELLS (8)

◯◯◯◯◯◯◯◯

4 HINTING TOLL (7, 4)

◯◯◯◯◯◯◯ ◯◯◯◯

5 TWENTY OR MAP (6, 5)

⬜⬜⬜⬜⬜⬜ ⬜⬜⬜⬜⬜

6 DODGY HOUR NAG (9, 3)

⬜⬜⬜⬜⬜⬜⬜⬜⬜
⬜⬜⬜

7 ODD GIRL IN SOS (7, 5)

⬜⬜⬜⬜⬜⬜⬜
⬜⬜⬜⬜⬜

8 STEALTH LASH (4, 3, 4)

⬜⬜⬜⬜ ⬜⬜⬜
⬜⬜⬜⬜

9 ABSENT THEM (3, 4, 3)

⬜⬜⬜ ⬜⬜⬜⬜
⬜⬜⬜

10 DREDGE NEW INSIGHT (3, 7, 6)

⬜⬜⬜ ⬜⬜⬜⬜⬜⬜⬜
⬜⬜⬜⬜⬜⬜

Answers on page 118

CROSSWORD 3

Solve the clues and discover the
1990s anagram in the shaded boxes!

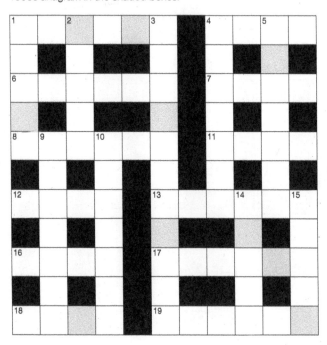

Across
1 Leave suddenly (6)
4 Stinging insect (4)
6 Womb resident (6)
7 Tenant's payment to a landlord (4)
8 Curved fruit (6)
11 Excitement (4)
12 Cougar (4)
13 Loads (6)
16 Mix (4)
17 Frozen water drops (6)
18 Con (4)
19 Annually (6)

Down
1 Nerd (5)
2 Private room on a ship (5)
3 Likelihood (11)
4 Combat vessel (7)
5 Child's play container (7)
9 Relating to water (7)
10 Set of rearranged letters (7)
14 Open sore (5)
15 Grotty (5)

Solution on page 131

OUR BEDROOM DECOR ESSENTIALS

Bean bag	Floating candles	Magic eye
Beanie bears	Forever friends	Posters
Border	Hi-fi	Sunflowers
Discman	Inflatable chair	Sun moon stars
Dreamcatcher	Lava lamp	Windchime

```
N  I  F  I  R  S  I  S  R  L  T  P  S  S  C
S  N  L  S  Y  I  E  S  A  G  M  F  M  N  L
R  F  O  N  R  Y  F  C  I  A  B  O  R  L  I
E  L  A  S  I  E  N  I  L  S  E  R  A  T  R
W  A  T  U  S  A  T  A  H  R  A  E  B  U  E
O  T  I  N  R  O  V  S  F  H  N  V  M  I  H
L  A  N  M  N  A  L  E  O  S  I  E  A  O  C
F  B  G  O  L  D  H  M  W  P  E  R  G  M  T
N  L  C  O  H  I  R  I  G  B  B  F  I  A  A
U  E  A  N  G  S  E  H  A  E  E  R  C  T  C
S  C  N  S  E  C  D  C  W  A  A  I  E  U  M
E  H  D  T  S  M  R  D  T  N  R  E  Y  D  A
T  A  L  A  D  A  O  N  L  B  S  N  E  A  E
F  I  E  R  H  N  B  I  B  A  C  D  G  N  R
F  R  S  S  O  R  L  W  N  G  B  S  A  S  D
```

Solution on page 121

COLOUR TIME

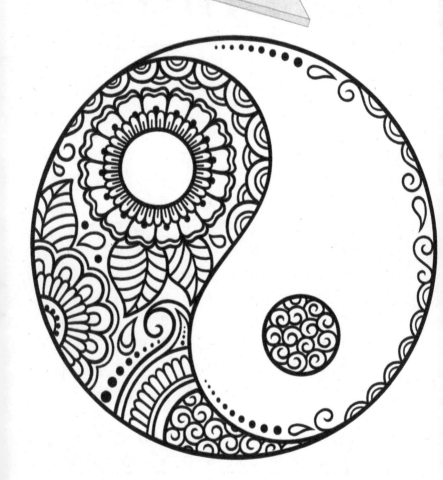

CROSSWORD 4

Solve the clues and discover the 1990s anagram in the shaded boxes!

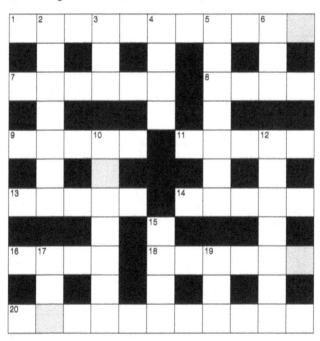

Across

1 The state of being a subject of a country (11)
7 Broad, city road (6)
8 Egg-laying location (4)
9 Elegance (5)
11 Transparent (5)
13 Denim legwear (5)
14 Mentally prepare; excite (5)
16 Atoll (4)
18 Loathing (6)
20 Lack of ability (11)

Down

2 Reciprocal (7)
3 Charged atom (3)
4 At any time (4)
5 Ones (7)
6 All the details: ___ and outs (3)
10 Not allow to be seen (7)
12 Speech patterns (7)
15 Used to identify a specific item (4)
17 Bro's opposite (3)
19 Metal container (3)

Solution on page 132

SWEET VALLEY HIGH

Aaron Dallas
Alice
Bruce Patman
Cheerleader
Elizabeth
Enid Rollins
Francine Pascal

Gladiators
Jessica
Library
Lila Fowler
Ned
Pi Beta Alpha
Steven

The Oracle
Todd Wilkins
Twins
Unicorn Club
Wakefield
Winston Egbert

```
L C E N I D R O L L I N S A E
S A H E L C A R O E H T L S U
C N C E A J W D N C S I A R N
B D I S E A E N N T C L E E I
R L Y K A R R S E E L L L L C
U E R L L P L V S A D A I W O
C I A T F I E E D I A T Z O R
E F R I I N W N A P C R A F N
P E B E T I O D I D N A B A C
A K I N L R T E D C E W E L L
T A L I A L I A B O N R T I U
M W E A T W I N S S T A H L B
A W I N S T O N E G B E R T C
N W G L A D I A T O R S E F H
A A P I B E T A A L P H A B W
```

Solution on page 121

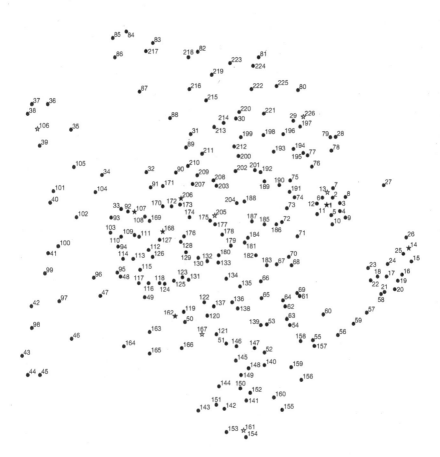

Recognise this classic children's book?

Draw straight lines to join the stars and dots in numerical order. Each time you reach a hollow star, lift your pen and continue drawing from the next solid star.

Solution on page 137

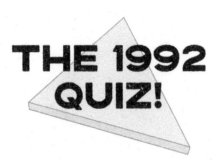

THE 1992 QUIZ!

1   Which cover of an old Dolly Parton song was used in a movie soundtrack in 1992, and held the record for the most number of weeks at number 1 in the UK singles charts until 2019?

2   Which iconic sneaker debuted in 1992 and sold 5 million pairs in this year?

3   Kris Kross, known for songs such as 'Jump', sparked which unusual style craze?

4   It was the twenty-fifth Olympic Games! Which city and country hosted in 1992?

5   What was the name of the colourless alternative to a popular mainstream fizzy drink released in 1992 and discontinued only two years later?

6   What was the bestselling Christmas toy in the USA this year?

7 In 1992, Kinder Surprise released a collection of ten small, green turtles to collect. What were they called?

8 Which male R&B group came to the 'end of the road' in 1992?

9 The first SMS text message ever sent was on 3 December 1992. What did it say?

10 Which comedy film coined the catchphrases 'Schwing!' and 'Party on!'?

Answers on page 116

THE GAMES WE GOT ADDICTED TO

Banjo Kazooie	Gran Turismo	Super Mario
Bust-A-Move	Lemmings	Tetris
Crash Bandicoot	Mortal Kombat	Theme Park
Donkey Kong	Resident Evil	The Oregon Trail
Earthworm Jim	Sim City	Tomb Raider
Grand Theft Auto	Sonic	Tony Hawks

T	O	O	C	I	D	N	A	B	H	S	A	R	C	T
O	L	S	U	P	E	R	M	A	R	I	O	N	L	O
R	T	I	T	M	L	E	M	M	I	N	G	S	I	B
E	G	U	A	O	E	K	M	O	S	M	O	K	V	A
A	R	E	A	R	M	S	O	N	I	C	M	W	E	N
R	A	S	G	T	T	B	E	A	T	T	A	A	T	J
T	N	B	N	A	F	N	R	L	E	S	S	H	N	O
H	T	U	O	L	S	E	O	A	N	A	B	Y	E	K
W	U	S	K	K	I	T	H	G	I	A	R	N	D	A
O	R	T	Y	O	M	A	E	T	E	D	I	O	I	Z
R	I	A	E	M	C	E	T	T	D	R	E	T	S	O
M	S	M	K	B	I	M	T	E	R	N	O	R	E	O
J	M	O	N	A	T	K	I	W	B	I	A	E	R	I
I	O	V	O	T	Y	R	R	D	T	D	S	R	H	E
M	I	E	D	T	H	E	M	E	P	A	R	K	G	T

Solution on page 122

CROSSWORD 5

Solve the clues and discover the
1990s anagram in the shaded boxes!

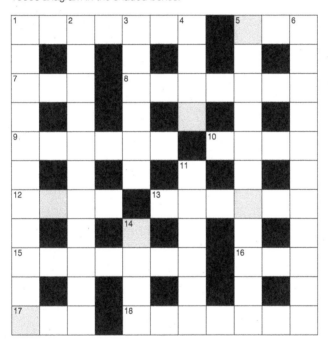

Across

1 Average (7)
5 Go bad (3)
7 Earlier (3)
8 Enduring artistic work (7)
9 Noises (6)
10 Japanese wheat noodles (4)
12 Made things up (4)
13 Wry (6)
15 At the shortest distance (7)
16 Ailing (3)
17 Regular drunkard (3)
18 Inherent mental ability (7)

Down

1 Organ donation ops (11)
2 Bulging (11)
3 Noisy grass insect (6)
4 Uncut bread (4)
5 Designed to be lived in (11)
6 Strictly; according to the facts (11)
11 Arts journalist, perhaps (6)
14 Unable to hear (4)

Solution on page 132

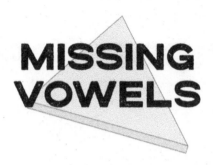

Iconic albums

All of the vowels have been removed from the names of these classic 1990s albums and the bands or singers who recorded them. Can you restore them?

1 NVRMND by NRVN

_____

2 K CMPTR by RDHD

_____

3 RSNBL DBT by JY-Z

_____

4 GRC by JFF BCKLY

_____

5 DK by GRN DY

_____

6 TH SLM SHDY LP by MNM

_____

7 WHT'S TH STRY MRNNG GLRY by SS

_____

8 TH SCR by FGS

_____

9 JGGD LTTL PLL by LNS MRSSTT

_____

10 TH GHST F TM JD by BRC SPRNGSTN

_____

Answers on page 118

THE SITCOMS
WE WATCHED
EVERY WEEK

Ally McBeal	Frasier	Moesha
Blossom	Fresh Prince	Seinfeld
Boy Meets World	Friends	Sex and the City
Buffy	Full House	Sister
Dinosaurs	Home Improvement	Spin City
Ellen	Kenan And Kel	Teen Angel

```
S  E  X  A  N  D  T  H  E  C  I  T  Y  H  V
B  L  D  E  Y  B  V  O  S  E  N  A  C  F  E
S  P  I  L  S  T  D  L  E  F  N  I  E  S  S
D  S  N  B  R  U  I  E  O  E  N  O  S  M  R
N  A  O  N  L  O  O  C  N  P  M  E  D  O  E
E  Y  S  E  S  O  W  H  N  B  E  F  P  E  I
I  R  A  B  L  R  S  S  L  I  U  D  E  S  S
R  O  U  C  A  A  P  S  T  L  P  F  T  H  A
F  H  R  E  T  S  I  S  O  E  U  S  F  A  R
A  L  S  L  L  S  R  E  T  M  E  F  A  Y  F
H  O  M  E  I  M  P  R  O  V  E  M  E  N  T
L  E  K  D  N  A  N  A  N  E  K  T  Y  N  N
T  E  E  N  A  N  G  E  L  L  E  N  E  O  U
N  I  N  E  C  N  I  R  P  H  S  E  R  F  B
E  T  A  L  L  Y  M  C  B  E  A  L  K  S  A
```

Solution on page 122

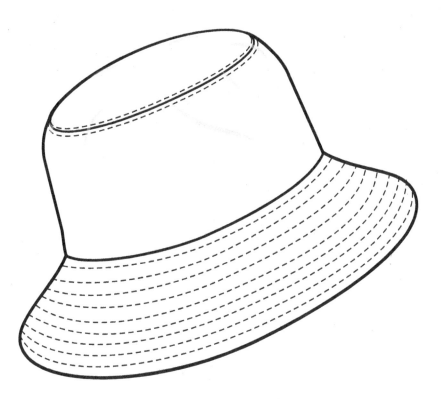

COLOUR TIME

CROSSWORD
6

Solve the clues and discover the 1990s anagram in the shaded boxes!

Across
1 Knowledgeable people (11)
7 Cow's low (3)
8 Least shallow (7)
9 Loan (4)
10 More concise (6)
13 Published (6)
14 Mathematical positions (4)
16 Upgrade (7)
18 Decorative knot in a ribbon (3)
19 Not specialized (11)

Down
1 Moaning (11)
2 Basis (7)
3 Chances (4)
4 Masticated (6)
5 Original surname (3)
6 Questioned (11)
11 Celebrity life (7)
12 Diversion (6)
15 Underground water source (4)
17 Cooking dish (3)

Solution on page 132

1990s MUSIC ICONS

Britney Spears
Celine Dion
Coolio
George Michael
Gloria Estefan
Janet Jackson
Jennifer Lopez

Jon Bon Jovi
Lauren Hill
Lisa Loeb
Madonna
Mariah Carey
Meat Loaf
Montell Jordan

Paula Abdul
Ricky Martin
Seal
Toni Braxton
Usher
Vanilla Ice

M	O	N	T	E	L	L	J	O	R	D	A	N	B	L
O	Z	T	V	E	L	A	O	M	N	C	J	Y	R	E
T	E	G	N	A	F	I	E	I	E	T	E	C	I	A
O	P	L	L	E	N	A	S	L	R	H	J	T	H
N	O	L	G	O	T	I	I	A	A	O	A	E	N	C
I	L	U	L	L	R	N	L	C	L	N	O	J	E	I
B	R	M	O	I	E	I	H	L	E	O	O	C	Y	M
R	E	A	A	D	H	A	A	T	A	N	E	R	S	E
A	F	O	I	D	I	N	J	E	B	I	E	B	P	G
X	I	O	S	R	O	A	E	O	S	H	C	A	E	R
T	N	A	A	E	C	N	N	R	S	T	A	E	A	O
O	N	M	F	K	A	J	N	U	U	O	E	E	R	E
N	E	T	S	E	O	L	E	A	U	A	E	F	S	G
I	J	O	L	V	L	U	D	B	A	A	L	U	A	P
N	N	N	I	T	R	A	M	Y	K	C	I	R	A	N

Solution on page 123

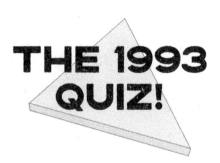

THE 1993 QUIZ!

1 Which movie franchise, directed by Steven Spielberg, began in 1993?

2 What is the name of the collectible cuddly toy line that was created in 1993 and included Legs the Frog, Flash the Dolphin and the highly sought-after, royal-blue version of Peanut the Elephant?

3 Which star performed at the halftime show at the Super Bowl in 1993?

4 In October 1993, actor River Phoenix died of drug-induced heart failure on the sidewalk outside which West Hollywood nightclub?

5 Which female tennis player won three grand slams this year?

6 Which sitcom that had premiered in 1982 aired its last show in May 1993, to huge viewing figures?

7 Which digital encyclopaedia program was initially released on CD-ROM in 1993?

8 Which of the following shows began in 1993?

   a) *Friends*

   b) *ER*

   c) *The X-Files*

   d) *The Fresh Prince of Bel-Air*

9 Which sitcom introduced us to Cory, his older brother Eric, younger sister Morgan and his neighbour and teacher Mr Feeny?

10 Which basketball player shocked the world when he decided to retire and pursue a career in professional baseball instead?

Answers on page 116

THE NEW ADVENTURES OF SUPERMAN

Cape	Jimmy Olsen	Newspaper
Clark Kent	Kryptonite	Secret identity
Daily Planet	Lane Smith	Smallville
Dean Cain	Lex Luthor	Superhero
Earth	Lois Lane	Teri Hatcher
Glasses	Metropolis	Villain

```
E  E  T  I  Y  T  L  E  X  L  U  T  H  O  R
U  T  N  E  K  K  R  A  L  C  E  I  Y  H  L
T  I  I  T  G  S  U  V  K  N  S  C  T  E  S
S  S  E  N  I  L  I  R  A  L  E  R  I  L  M
N  O  I  N  O  L  A  L  S  N  A  L  T  N  A
E  I  T  L  L  T  P  S  A  E  A  E  N  E  L
W  I  L  A  O  Y  P  L  S  N  V  D  E  S  L
S  R  I  C  L  P  S  Y  E  E  R  E  D  L  V
P  N  A  I  E  I  O  S  R  R  S  A  I  O  I
A  D  A  K  O  P  M  R  E  K  T  N  T  Y  L
P  D  E  L  N  I  A  L  T  N  L  C  E  M  L
E  I  E  I  T  R  T  C  E  E  O  A  R  M  E
R  A  E  H  S  S  O  A  T  E  M  I  C  I  T
R  E  H  C  T  A  H  I  R  E  T  N  E  J  L
E  L  S  U  P  E  R  H  E  R  O  R  S  R  A
```

Solution on page 123

CROSSWORD 7

Solve the clues and discover the 1990s anagram in the shaded boxes!

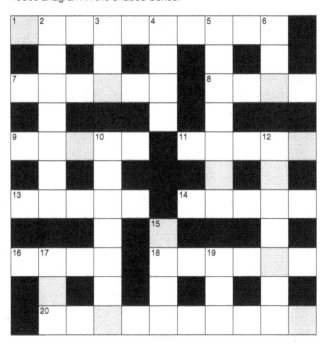

Across
1 Music from a movie (10)
7 Dominions (6)
8 Cut (4)
9 Widespread destruction (5)
11 Rustic paradise (5)
13 Baton race (5)
14 Thoughts (5)
16 Bean curd (4)
18 Beat (6)
20 Belittling (10)

Down
2 Run (7)
3 Nada (3)
4 Long, pointed tooth (4)
5 Averted (7)
6 Japanese carp (3)
10 Less transparent (7)
12 Cured animal skin (7)
15 Boast (4)
17 Elderly (3)
19 Even so (3)

Solution on page 133

SAVED BY THE BELL

AC Slater	Kevin	Time Out
Basketball	Lisa Turtle	Valley High
Bayside High	Mascot	Violet
Cheerleader	Mr Belding	Zack Attack
Homecoming	Screech	Zack Morris
Jessie Spano	The Max	
Kelly Kapowski	Tiger	

```
E C H E E R L E A D E R K E R
N E K R C L L A B T E K S A B
T T E D L S I R R O M K C A Z
I J L M H G O X A M E H T J E
H E L A B G N I D L E B R M L
O S Y Z K A I C T U O E M I T
M S K G A A Y H L H C E O Z R
E I A E S C E S Y K E H S I U
C E P C V T K H I E E C K Y T
O S O R S E T A C D L V D M A
M P W L A L A O T E E L I D S
I A S U O O A I C T E H A N I
N N K I C I R T K S A R I V L
G O I E I V T A E G A C C G M
T L V K S T I G E R E M K S H
```

Solution on page 123

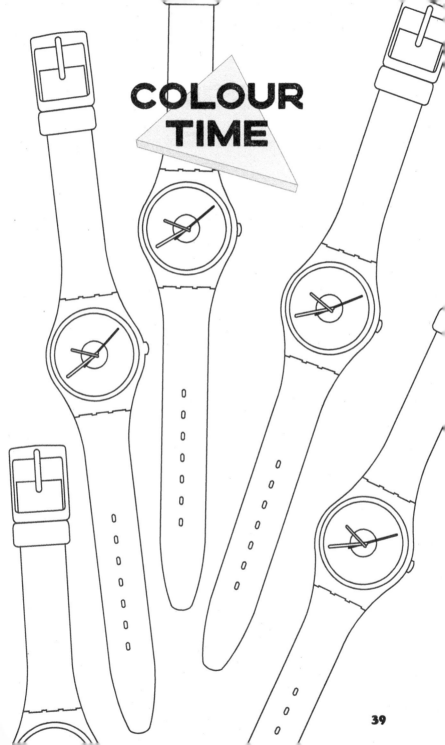

COLOUR TIME

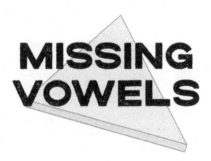

MISSING VOWELS

The Most-Watched *X-Files* Episodes

Mulder and Scully landed on our screens in 1993 and kept us believing in aliens for nine consecutive seasons. All of the vowels have been removed from the names of the series' most-watched episodes. Can you restore them?

1 LNRD BTTS

_____

2 RDX

_____

3 DTR

_____

4 NSL SSPCTS

_____

5 SCHZGNY

_____

6 NVR GN

_____

7 TH RN KNG

_____

8 TH SXTH XTNCTN

_____

9 FRSH BNS

_____

10 SMLL PTTS

_____

Answers on page 119

Draw straight lines to join the stars and dots in numerical order. Each time you reach a hollow star, lift your pen and continue drawing from the next solid star.

Solution on page 138

42

When Shakespeare suddenly got a whole lot more interesting

CROSSWORD 8

Solve the clues and discover the
1990s anagram in the shaded boxes!

Across
1 Secret sequences (9)
8 Do very well (5)
9 Cults (5)
10 Loftier (6)
12 Large, cruel giant (4)
14 Mosque prayer leader (4)
15 Merged (6)
17 Existing (5)
18 Mountain ash (5)
20 This puzzle (9)

Down
2 Curve (3)
3 Figured out (6)
4 Drive out; expel (4)
5 Ten-sided polygon (7)
6 Specialized (9)
7 Rising (9)
11 Slow-moving mass of ice (7)
13 Take from a library (6)
16 Spiders' homes (4)
19 State of armed combat (3)

Solution on page 133

THE BOOKS WE LOVED AS TEENS

Adrian Mole
Anastasia
Babysitters Club
Cafe Club
Girl Talk
Goggle Eyes

Goosebumps
Judy Blume
Making Out
Mary Bubnik
Nancy Drew
Point Horror

Point Romance
Sweet Dreams
The Party Line
Toning the Sweep

B	U	L	C	S	R	E	T	T	I	S	Y	B	A	B
O	N	E	B	O	E	I	E	M	E	T	E	C	T	A
R	K	I	N	T	M	T	J	Y	G	C	Y	A	U	D
O	L	S	N	I	R	A	E	B	N	O	T	F	O	R
R	A	R	P	O	L	E	R	A	R	J	G	E	G	I
R	T	O	A	M	L	Y	M	Y	U	N	N	C	N	A
O	L	N	A	G	U	O	T	D	B	A	P	L	I	N
H	R	T	G	N	R	B	Y	R	N	U	L	U	K	M
T	I	O	E	T	A	B	E	C	A	B	B	B	A	O
N	G	S	N	B	L	S	Y	S	B	P	M	N	M	L
I	I	I	B	U	D	D	T	B	O	B	E	Y	I	E
O	O	I	M	G	R	A	T	A	T	O	S	H	T	K
P	E	E	G	E	N	R	A	H	S	N	G	B	T	B
P	E	E	W	S	E	H	T	G	N	I	N	O	T	M
K	M	P	S	W	E	E	T	D	R	E	A	M	S	M

Solution on page 124

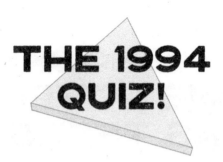

THE 1994 QUIZ!

1 Which brand's 'Hello Boys' campaign from 1994 is considered one of the most iconic ads of all time?

2 This was the year that rock music lost Kurt Cobain. Who was he married to?

3 What was the highest grossing film of 1994?

4 Australian drama *Heartbreak High* hit the screens with the love affair between Jodie Cooper and Nick Poulus gripping viewers. However, Nick died at the end of series one, leaving a distraught Jodie. How did Nick die?

5 *My So-Called Life* aired in 1994 and was critically praised for its realistic portrayal of adolescence. Set at the fictional Liberty High School in Pennsylvania, it follows the lives of a group of teenagers with the central character played by Claire Danes. What was the character's name?

6 Which English actor and model famously wore a black Versace dress held together by oversized gold safety pins when she accompanied her then-boyfriend to the premiere of *Four Weddings and a Funeral* in 1994?

7 Which of the following pop stars did not begin their career as a cast member on *The All New Mickey Mouse Club*?

a) Britney Spears
b) Justin Timberlake
c) Christina Aguilera
d) Miley Cyrus
e) Ryan Gosling

8 In the 1994 movie *Pulp Fiction*, what did John Travolta's character inform us a quarter pounder with cheese is called in France?

9 What were the names of the twins in the hit sitcom *Sister, Sister*?

10 Which movie character likened life to a box of chocolates?

Answers on pages 116–117

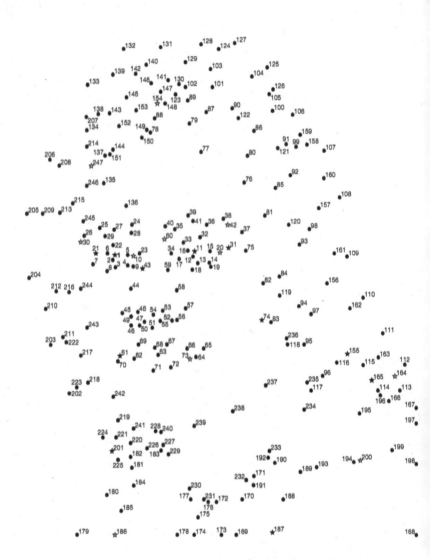

Star of *My So-Called Life* and every thinking girl's heartthrob

Draw straight lines to join the stars and dots in numerical order.
Each time you reach a hollow star, lift your pen and
continue drawing from the next solid star.

Solution on page 138

1990s
BLOCKBUSTER
MOVIES

Armageddon	Good Will Hunting	Pulp Fiction
Austin Powers	Home Alone	Romeo And Juliet
Batman Forever	Independence Day	Speed
Braveheart	Jumanji	Toy Story
Casper	Jurassic Park	Twister
Clueless	Liar Liar	Wayne's World
Forrest Gump	Men In Black	

```
R  E  V  E  R  O  F  N  A  M  T  A  B  I  G
J  T  W  P  U  L  P  F  I  C  T  I  O  N  L
U  E  M  A  C  L  U  E  L  E  S  S  I  D  S
R  I  E  L  Y  R  O  T  S  Y  O  T  R  E  R
A  L  N  I  J  N  A  M  U  J  N  S  N  P  E
S  U  I  A  R  O  E  I  S  U  P  O  P  E  W
S  J  N  R  E  E  M  S  H  P  L  P  R  N  O
I  D  B  L  I  D  T  L  W  A  E  E  A  D  P
C  N  L  I  P  O  L  S  E  O  P  E  R  E  N
P  A  A  A  T  I  U  M  I  S  R  V  D  N  I
A  O  C  R  W  N  O  O  A  W  S  L  O  C  T
R  E  K  D  G  H  O  C  P  S  T  E  D  E  S
K  M  O  A  R  M  A  G  E  D  D  O  N  D  U
T  O  F  O  R  R  E  S  T  G  U  M  P  A  A
G  R  B  R  A  V  E  H  E  A  R  T  A  Y  I
```

Solution on page 124

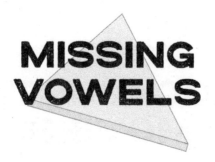

Sports Stars

All of the vowels have been removed from the
names of these iconic 1990s sportspeople.
Can you restore them?

1 MCHL JRDN

_____

2 NDR GSS

_____

3 SRN WLLMS

_____

4 SHQLL 'NL

_____

5 RNLD

_____

6 BRTT FVR

_____

7 M HMM

_____

8 MKE TYSN

_____

9 MCHLL KWN

_____

10 RC CNTN

_____

Answers on page 119

CROSSWORD 9

Solve the clues and discover the
1990s anagram in the shaded boxes!

Across
1 Was of the correct size (6)
4 Furniture for sleeping on (4)
6 Red gems (6)
7 Diplomacy (4)
8 Mixed cereal breakfast (6)
11 Periods of history (4)
12 Post-larval insect (4)
13 Old Faithful, eg (6)
16 Unable to feel (4)
17 Bring in from abroad (6)
18 Contract a muscle (4)
19 Domiciled (6)

Down
1 Roman marketplace (5)
2 Flat-topped furniture item (5)
3 Tell the difference (11)
4 Voltaic cell (7)
5 Read aloud for transcription (7)
9 Strange; rare (7)
10 Crate used for speaking from (7)
14 Sales outlets (5)
15 Gave five stars, perhaps (5)

Solution on page 133

THE PMs AND PRESIDENTS OF THE 1990s

Blair
Bolger
Brown
Bush
Campbell
Chretien

Clark
Clinton
Hawke
Howard
Keating
Major

Moore
Mulroney
Palmer
Shipley
Thatcher

E	H	C	A	P	N	H	B	B	L	H	E	S	R	E
B	A	L	L	O	I	E	K	L	U	N	A	B	R	A
L	A	M	U	L	R	O	N	E	Y	S	M	L	E	L
A	H	G	E	R	O	O	M	E	A	S	H	M	M	L
E	O	L	E	E	H	B	L	M	E	T	D	N	L	E
R	W	B	H	G	O	I	M	T	K	R	I	G	A	B
P	A	W	P	L	D	E	D	R	L	R	U	N	P	P
T	R	E	E	O	J	R	A	T	R	O	E	O	G	M
W	D	R	O	B	U	L	H	A	L	J	M	H	H	A
B	A	I	R	C	C	A	A	T	N	A	B	N	A	C
B	O	A	O	U	T	K	N	A	R	M	L	P	W	E
R	B	L	H	C	A	N	O	T	N	I	L	C	K	H
O	S	B	H	N	E	I	T	E	R	H	C	A	E	M
W	P	E	P	Y	E	L	P	I	H	S	T	B	B	S
N	R	G	R	J	B	E	A	R	K	R	T	A	K	R

Solution on page 124

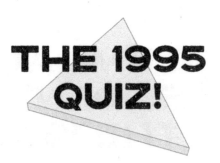

THE 1995 QUIZ!

1   Two rival British bands were in the 'Battle of
    Britpop' in 1995 when they released singles on the
    same day. What were the bands and what were the
    names of their singles?

2   Pamela Anderson married which Mötley Crüe
    drummer on a beach in Mexico?

3   Which popstar announced they would be leaving
    which band in 1995, breaking the hearts of teens
    all over the world?

4   In 1995 the first blue M&M made its appearance.
    What colour did it replace?

5   Alicia Silverstone was propelled to fame in *Clueless*.
    What term was used in the movie to describe a
    'handsome or gorgeous man'?

6   Which online dating service launched in this year?

7   Pizza Hut debuted which style of pizza in 1995?

8 The televised trial of which ex-football player accused of killing his ex-wife captivated the world during 1995?

9 We were all obsessed with learning the lyrics to which rapper's Grammy-winning song after it was featured in the movie *Dangerous Minds*?

10 What was the first feature film to have a fully CGI character in a leading role?

Answers on page 117

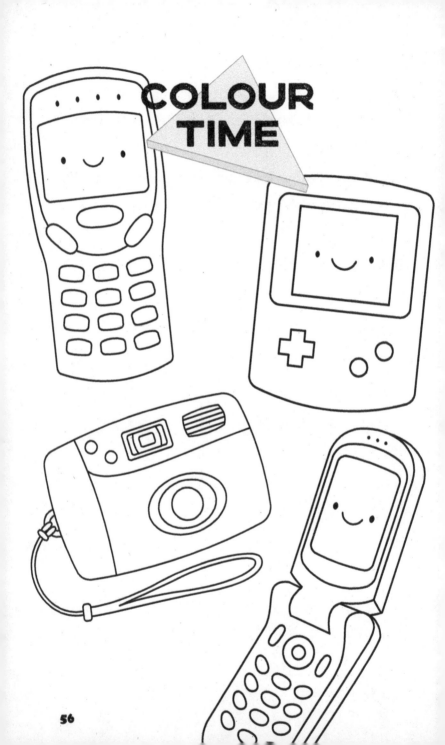

COLOUR
TIME

THE SNACKS AND DRINKS WE ENJOYED

Cheez Balls
Cosmopolitan
Dunkeroos
Fruit Winders
Hawaiian Punch
Hubba Bubba
Jolly Ranchers

Lunchables
Nerds
Ouch! Bubblegum
Pez
Pop Tarts
Push Pop
Rainbow Drops

Red Bull
Sarah Lee
Space Raiders
Sunny Delight
Tab Clear
Vice Versas

E	S	R	E	D	N	I	W	T	I	U	R	F	D	V
B	H	A	W	A	I	I	A	N	P	U	N	C	H	E
O	E	S	P	A	C	E	R	A	I	D	E	R	S	C
T	U	S	R	E	H	C	N	A	R	Y	L	L	O	J
A	H	C	N	A	T	I	L	O	P	O	M	S	O	C
V	L	G	H	A	I	E	O	D	P	L	N	H	R	C
I	U	S	I	B	B	N	E	S	E	S	A	T	E	R
C	N	T	L	L	U	B	B	L	Z	U	A	U	K	A
E	C	R	S	L	E	B	U	O	H	B	R	F	N	E
V	H	A	D	W	U	D	B	B	W	A	G	A	U	L
E	A	T	R	E	S	B	Y	L	A	D	R	L	D	C
R	B	P	E	A	O	U	D	N	E	B	R	A	I	B
S	L	O	N	B	A	B	S	E	N	G	B	O	S	A
A	E	P	O	P	H	S	U	P	R	U	U	U	P	T
S	S	L	L	A	B	Z	E	E	H	C	S	M	H	S

Solution on page 125

CROSSWORD 10

Solve the clues and discover the
1990s anagram in the shaded boxes!

Across
1 Assigned (9)
7 Summarize (5)
8 Nut from an oak tree (5)
10 Opposite of pro (4)
11 Area cast into partial darkness (6)
14 Absolute truth (6)
15 Basis for cheese (4)
17 Bordered (5)
19 Spiky-leaved plant (5)
20 Environs (9)

Down
2 Finds (7)
3 Accident exclamation (4)
4 Indifference (6)
5 The self (3)
6 Metal percussion instrument (8)
9 In the present era (8)
12 Twofold (7)
13 Perform (6)
16 You (archaic) (4)
18 Large, dark antelope (3)

Solution on page 134

OUR BEAUTY MUST-HAVES

Angel dust
Apricot scrub
Bath beads
Blue eyeshadow
Body glitter
Bronzing pearls
CK One

Crimping iron
Exclamation
Hair mascara
Hard Candy
Herbal Essences
Hot oil
Impulse

Lip Smackers
Lynx
Sun-In
Tommy Girl
Wash and Go
White Musk

S	I	Y	O	N	O	I	T	A	M	A	L	C	X	E
S	E	B	U	R	C	S	T	O	C	I	R	P	A	R
W	L	C	C	H	S	R	L	N	N	O	I	L	Y	E
H	H	R	N	R	R	U	X	N	Y	L	G	I	D	T
A	Y	I	A	E	I	O	N	H	A	E	Y	O	N	T
I	T	W	T	E	S	M	G	I	L	I	M	T	A	I
R	T	P	Y	E	P	S	P	D	N	E	M	O	C	L
M	P	E	Z	G	M	G	E	I	N	O	O	H	D	G
A	C	K	O	N	E	U	N	L	N	A	T	H	R	Y
S	E	H	N	A	U	T	S	I	A	G	H	R	A	D
C	I	M	P	U	L	S	E	K	Z	B	I	S	H	O
A	B	A	T	H	B	E	A	D	S	N	R	R	A	B
R	A	N	G	E	L	D	U	S	T	E	O	E	O	W
A	L	I	P	S	M	A	C	K	E	R	S	R	H	N
B	L	U	E	E	Y	E	S	H	A	D	O	W	B	O

Solution on page 125

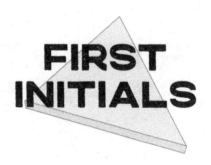

FIRST INITIALS

Horror Movies

Can you work out which 90s horror films that scared the bejesus out of us have been clued below, where only the initials of each film's title have been given? *Edward Scissorhands*, for example, would be given as 'E S'.

1 I K W Y D L S

_____

2 T S O T L

_____

3 T B W P

_____

4 T P U T S

_____

5 T H T R T C

_____

6 I W T V

_____

7 W C N N

_____

8 T S S

_____

9 B S D

_____

10 I

_____

Answers on page 119

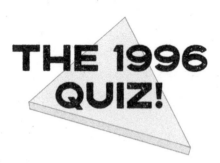

THE 1996 QUIZ!

1 Which song did duo Los del Rio have a hit with this year?

2 The Cardigans' 'Lovefool' featured in which hit 1996 movie?

3 This year marked the beginning of the *Scream* horror series. How many murders were there in the first movie?

4 The Fugees released *The Score* this year. Can you name all three members?

5 In the *Friends* episode entitled 'The One at the Beach', Rachel encourages Ross's girlfriend Bonnie to do what?

6 In 1996, scientists successfully cloned a mammal for the first time via the process of somatic cell nuclear transfer. What was the name given to the animal?

7 Which internet search engine launched in 1996?

8 What 1996 movie featured Michael Jordan and the Looney Tunes?

9 Which creepy movie got us playing 'light as a feather, stiff as a board'?

10 Which singer's daughter, Lourdes, was born in October 1996?

Answers on page 117

If you were a child in the 1990s you probably owned one of these

Draw straight lines to join the stars and dots in numerical order. Each time you reach a hollow star, lift your pen and continue drawing from the next solid star.

Solution on page 139

POPULAR NAMES IN THE 1990s

Abigail	Jacob	Nathan
Bethany	Jessica	Oliver
Chloe	Jodie	Reece
Connor	Jordan	Samuel
Dylan	Kirsty	Sophie
Elliot	Melissa	Stephanie
Harriet	Natashia	

S	S	L	J	H	E	N	J	O	D	I	E	N	C	L
T	A	H	I	E	R	P	O	E	E	A	E	O	T	I
J	C	C	K	A	S	E	C	O	N	N	O	R	A	K
N	K	S	I	O	G	S	B	R	J	A	C	O	B	N
A	R	C	R	Y	I	I	I	E	E	S	M	O	A	J
T	E	R	S	T	R	A	B	C	T	K	L	T	H	J
H	V	A	T	S	S	H	C	A	A	H	A	L	C	T
A	I	E	Y	S	G	E	E	L	R	S	A	H	D	T
N	L	L	I	I	I	A	S	I	H	R	L	N	A	S
L	O	L	I	T	E	I	L	I	N	O	E	M	Y	A
T	E	I	R	R	A	H	A	A	E	H	A	E	E	M
M	O	O	V	S	T	E	P	H	A	N	I	E	C	U
A	K	T	A	T	D	E	E	A	A	O	R	E	N	E
L	E	D	Y	L	A	N	O	E	C	L	T	S	M	L
Y	S	O	P	H	I	E	J	O	R	D	A	N	H	O

Solution on page 125

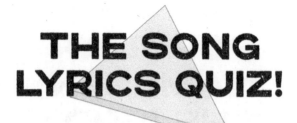

THE SONG LYRICS QUIZ!

1 Who played her enemies like a game of chess?

2 Who woke up in her make-up and decided it was too early for that dress?

3 Who wanted to be a little bit taller, have a rabbit in a hat and a girl who looked good?

4 Who wanted to know if they were your fire and your one desire?

5 Which Danish act promised to make you hers and take you to the top (pretty baby)?

6 Who proved slightly woolly on the definition of irony?

7 Who wanted to meet up in the year 2000 when we're all fully grown?

8 Where might you get to on Venga Airways?

9 Who didn't ever want to feel like he did that day?

10 Who bought his first real six-string in 1969?

11 Who wanted to clear it up if you seemed to be confused, because it's time we got this straight?

12 Who reckoned you should just say what you say without letting anyone get in your way?

Answers on page 117

CROSSWORD
11

Solve the clues and discover the
1990s anagram in the shaded boxes!

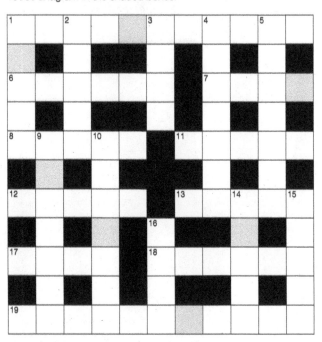

Across
1 Those living somewhere (11)
6 Film with a soundtrack (6)
7 Platform for loading ships (4)
8 Large shop (5)
11 Thin columns of smoke (5)
12 Overhead (5)
13 Digression (5)
17 Legatee (4)
18 Shrub of the honeysuckle family (6)
19 Overlay (11)

Down
1 Tiny bits (5)
2 Greeting word (5)
3 Freezes over (4)
4 Finds not guilty (7)
5 Caught (7)
9 Vivid pictorial impression (7)
10 Change to the opposite direction (7)
14 House made of ice (5)
15 Make extremely happy (5)
16 South Asian dress (4)

Solution on page 134

FRIENDS GUEST STARS

Brad Pitt	Gary Oldman	Morgan Fairchild
Charlton Heston	Hank Azaria	Paul Rudd
Dakota Fanning	Helen Hunt	Robin Williams
Danny Devito	Jennifer Grey	Sean Penn
Denise Richards	Julia Roberts	Selma Blair
Elle Macpherson	Kathleen Turner	Susan Sarandon

```
D  C  N  A  M  D  L  O  Y  R  A  G  G  E  J
E  S  H  E  L  E  N  H  U  N  T  N  S  L  E
N  E  D  A  N  N  Y  D  E  V  I  T  O  L  N
I  L  A  I  R  A  Z  A  K  N  A  H  B  E  N
S  M  A  I  L  L  I  W  N  I  B  O  R  M  I
E  A  R  E  B  L  T  A  O  E  A  D  A  A  F
R  B  R  A  L  M  F  O  L  N  T  G  D  C  E
I  L  U  E  A  A  J  N  N  F  R  L  P  P  R
C  A  N  R  T  S  J  O  A  H  M  L  I  H  G
H  I  L  O  N  N  E  P  N  A  E  S  T  E  R
A  R  K  P  A  U  L  R  U  D  D  S  T  R  E
R  A  J  U  L  I  A  R  O  B  E  R  T  S  Y
D  L  I  H  C  R  I  A  F  N  A  G  R  O  M
S  S  U  S  A  N  S  A  R  A  N  D  O  N  N
I  R  E  N  R  U  T  N  E  E  L  H  T  A  K
```

Solution on page 126

CROSSWORD 12

Solve the clues and discover the
1990s anagram in the shaded boxes!

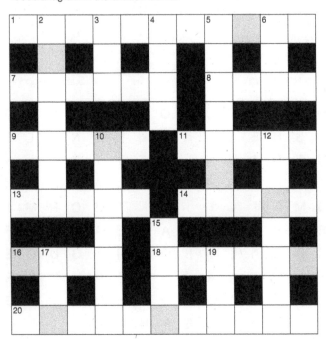

Across
1 Branch of philosophy (11)
7 Approve (6)
8 Picks, with 'for' (4)
9 Double-deckers, eg (5)
11 Stretch (5)
13 A show being broadcast again (5)
14 Bodily sacs (5)
16 Go without food (4)
18 Deliver a sermon (6)
20 Diminuendo (11)

Down
2 Keep out (7)
3 Affirmative vote (3)
4 Punches; strikes (4)
5 Soon (7)
6 Army bed (3)
10 Earth's midriff? (7)
12 Observed (7)
15 Set of musical works (4)
17 Very skilled person (3)
19 Vision organ (3)

Solution on page 134

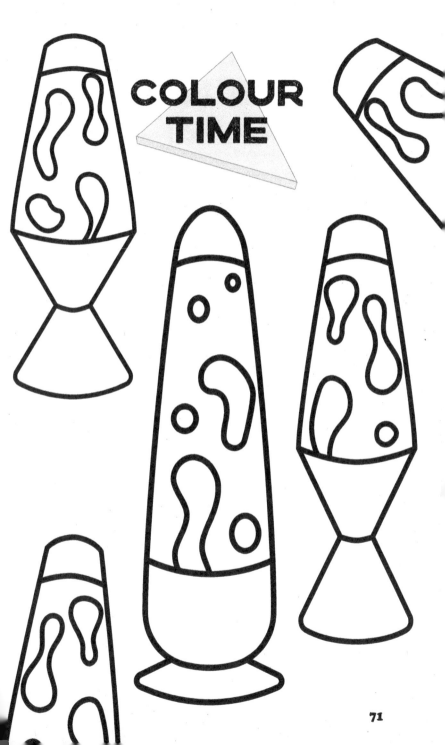

COLOUR TIME

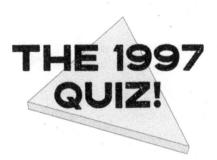

THE 1997 QUIZ!

1   Natalie Imbruglia left *Neighbours* and released her first single in 1997 – what was it called?

2   'Egg watch' is the English translation of the name of what popular toy released in the US and UK in 1997?

3   In 1997, Geri Halliwell announced she was leaving the Spice Girls. What year did she officially rejoin the group for a reunion tour?

4   Which three brothers released their earworm 'MMMBop' in 1997?

5   Which 1997 video was a parody of Michael Jackson's 'Thriller'?

6   Which four children's TV characters arrived on screen in 1997 with the catchphrase 'Eh oh!'?

7   Which film featured 'galaxy defenders' played by Will Smith and Tommy Lee Jones?

8 At the age of 14, who became the youngest person to ever win a Grammy?

9 'I'll Be Missing You', a song by American rapper Puff Daddy and singer Faith Evans, was written in memory of which artist?

10 Which actress came out as gay on her sitcom?

Answers on page 117

TOY STORY 1 AND 2

Alien
Andy
Barbie
Bo Peep
Bullseye
Buster
Buzz Lightyear

Emily
Jessie
Molly
Mr Potato Head
Mrs Davis
Sarge
Slinky Dog

Soldiers
Stinky Pete
The Cleaner
Wheezy
Woody
Zurg

P	S	B	A	R	B	I	E	U	S	A	R	G	E	G
T	S	Y	S	J	A	S	H	E	S	W	U	E	R	M
Y	B	T	U	R	A	L	M	O	H	S	G	U	G	Y
O	S	T	I	R	E	I	I	E	E	D	Z	O	R	D
A	P	M	H	N	L	I	E	E	P	A	D	O	E	O
H	E	E	A	Y	K	Z	D	L	N	Y	O	R	N	O
R	E	I	Y	S	Y	Y	G	L	K	D	E	Y	A	W
U	P	S	L	O	G	I	P	N	O	T	L	N	E	B
D	O	S	L	Y	B	S	I	E	S	S	D	L	L	U
L	B	E	O	Y	E	L	S	U	T	Y	L	I	C	L
T	R	J	M	C	S	E	B	B	T	E	L	L	E	L
M	M	R	P	O	T	A	T	O	H	E	A	D	H	S
A	U	I	A	S	I	V	A	D	S	R	M	O	T	E
S	E	U	R	C	N	G	E	Y	Y	E	E	I	A	Y
O	R	A	E	Y	T	H	G	I	L	Z	Z	U	B	E

Solution on page 126

CROSSWORD 13

Solve the clues and discover the
1990s anagram in the shaded boxes!

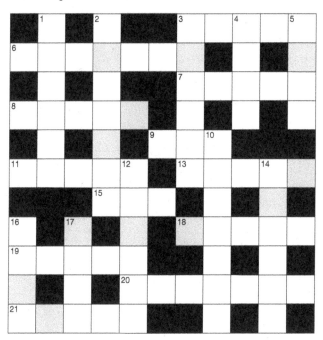

Across
3 Silver bar (5)
6 Essential growth nutrient (7)
7 Drops (5)
8 Speak (5)
9 Part of a play (3)
11 Dowdy woman (5)
13 Commerce (5)
15 Largest of all deer (3)
18 Sign of a fire (5)
19 Throw into confusion (5)
20 All-purpose (7)
21 Treat cruelly (5)

Down
1 Reflecting surface (6)
2 Combat period (7)
3 Contaminate (6)
4 18-hole game (4)
5 Chore (4)
10 Brass instrument (7)
12 Promise of a donation (6)
14 Authoritarian command (6)
16 Low-pitched musical instrument (4)
17 Sweetheart (4)

Solution on page 135

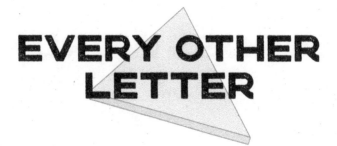

EVERY OTHER LETTER

Comedians

The people who made us LOL before we even knew what that meant! Restore the names of these 90s comedians by placing a letter into each gap.

1 ⬚ I ⬚ ⬚ C ⬚ R ⬚ E ⬚

2 C ⬚ R ⬚ S ⬚ O ⬚ K

3 D ⬚ V ⬚ ⬚ H ⬚ P ⬚ L ⬚ E

4 ⬚ D ⬚ M ⬚ S ⬚ N ⬚ L ⬚ R

5 M ⬚ R ⬚ A ⬚ E ⬚ ⬚ C ⬚ O

6 M ⬚ K ⬚ ⬚ Y ⬚ R ⬚

7 ☐ E ☐ R ☐
  S ☐ I ☐ F ☐ L ☐

8 ☐ T ☐ V ☐ H ☐ R ☐ E ☐

9 M ☐ R ☐ I ☐
  L ☐ W ☐ E ☐ C ☐

10 J ☐ A ☐ C ☐ L ☐ I ☐ S

Answers on page 119

THE FLOOR
FILLERS OF
THE 1990s

Baby One More Time
Believe
Bills Bills Bills
Black or White
Candle in the Wind
End of the Road
Genie in a Bottle

Ice Ice Baby
I'll Be Missing You
Kiss From a Rose
Mmmbop
My Heart Will Go On
No Scrubs
The Boy Is Mine

This Is How We Do It
Unbreak My Heart
Wannabe
Waterfalls
Wild Wild West

T	B	N	C	I	C	E	I	C	E	B	A	B	Y	T
E	I	O	A	L	T	I	K	E	V	T	W	A	D	R
L	L	O	N	L	E	E	I	B	E	H	I	B	A	A
T	L	G	D	B	A	T	S	A	I	E	L	Y	O	E
T	S	L	L	E	S	I	S	N	L	B	D	O	R	H
O	B	L	E	M	W	H	F	N	E	O	W	N	E	Y
B	I	I	I	I	A	W	R	A	B	Y	I	E	H	M
A	L	W	N	S	T	R	O	W	N	I	L	M	T	K
N	L	T	T	S	E	O	M	H	O	S	D	O	F	A
I	S	R	H	I	R	K	A	M	S	M	W	R	O	E
E	B	A	E	N	F	C	R	M	C	I	E	E	D	R
I	I	E	W	G	A	A	O	M	R	N	S	T	N	B
N	L	H	I	Y	L	L	S	B	U	E	T	I	E	N
E	L	Y	N	O	L	B	E	O	B	M	B	M	H	U
G	S	M	D	U	S	O	D	P	S	I	T	E	C	T

Solution on page 126

The ultimate strange 1990s collectible

Draw straight lines to join the stars and dots in numerical order. Each time you reach a hollow star, lift your pen and continue drawing from the next solid star.

Solution on page 139

79

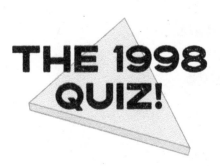

THE 1998 QUIZ!

1 Which sex toy grew in popularity after featuring in an episode of *Sex and the City* entitled 'The Turtle and the Hare'?

2 What was the most popular internet search engine in 1998?

3 In 1998 Starburst got their new name and branding in the UK, but what did they used to be called?

4 How many Oscars did *Titanic* win at the 1998 Academy Awards?

5 Which song was released as the lead single from album, *The Miseducation of Lauryn Hill* and debuted at number one on the Billboard Hot 100?

6 The school-set video for which 1998 song was voted by Billboard to be the best of the 1990s?

7 In which 1998 movie would you find the line: 'None of you have to go. We can all just sit here on Earth, wait for this big rock to crash into it, kill everything and everybody we know. United States government just asked us to save the world. Anybody wanna say no?'

8 In 1998 Brandy and Monica released hit single 'The Boy Is Mine', but which sitcom did Brandy rise to fame in?

9 Which song, released in 1998, was one of the first commercial recordings to feature the audio processor software Auto-Tune, used to produce the prominent altered effect on vocals?

10 Which British prime-time TV quiz show began in 1998 with the round 'fastest finger first' determining who got into the hot seat?

Answers on page 118

THE COOLEST 1990s DECOR

Artificial plant
Butterfly chair
CD cabinet
Chandelier
Curtain valance
Flower wallpaper

Frosted glass
Glass table
Green and purple
Neon sign
Pine furniture
Rope lights

Textured walls
Wallpaper border
Wall stencils
Wavy mirror
Wicker furniture

```
R  E  P  A  P  L  L  A  W  R  E  W  O  L  F
T  N  A  L  P  L  A  I  C  I  F  I  T  R  A
I  I  E  W  A  L  L  S  T  E  N  C  I  L  S
E  R  O  R  R  I  M  Y  V  A  W  K  E  N  N
E  L  P  R  U  P  D  N  A  N  E  E  R  G  G
G  L  A  S  S  T  A  B  L  E  I  R  O  W  I
S  S  A  L  G  D  E  T  S  O  R  F  G  L  S
T  R  E  I  L  E  D  N  A  H  C  U  U  A  N
E  C  N  A  L  A  V  N  I  A  T  R  U  C  O
R  O  P  E  L  I  G  H  T  S  N  N  C  A  E
E  R  U  T  I  N  R  U  F  E  N  I  P  F  N
P  R  I  A  H  C  Y  L  F  R  E  T  T  U  B
U  T  E  N  I  B  A  C  D  C  R  U  N  E  R
W  A  L  L  P  A  P  E  R  B  O  R  D  E  R
S  L  L  A  W  D  E  R  U  T  X  E  T  M  L
```

Solution on page 127

CROSSWORD 14

Solve the clues and discover the 1990s anagram in the shaded boxes!

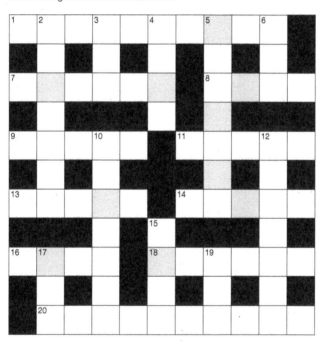

Across
1 Popular primula variety (10)
7 Infinitesimally small (6)
8 Mischievous children (4)
9 Award, perhaps (5)
11 Protective covering (5)
13 Ruin (5)
14 Practice (5)
16 Earthquake points of origin (4)
18 Adhere (6)
20 Open to bargaining (10)

Down
2 Surface rock formation (7)
3 A compliment to the chef? (3)
4 Bow notch (4)
5 Elevations (7)
6 Steep in liquid (3)
10 Apprehending; catching (7)
12 Reasoned (7)
15 Completely fascinated (4)
17 Confess to something: ___ up (3)
19 Brewed leaf drink (3)

Solution on page 135

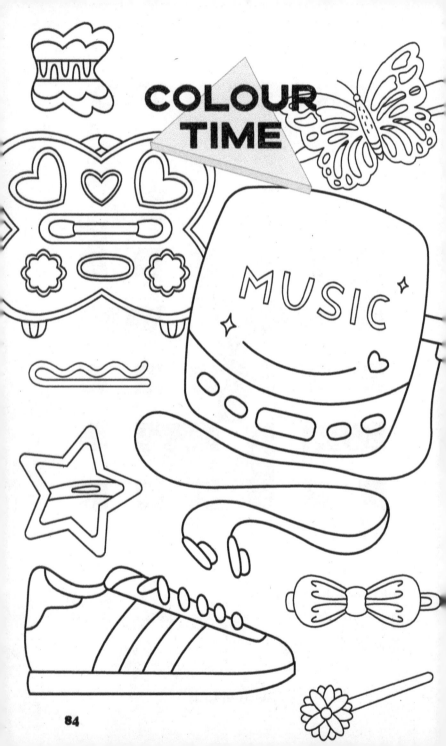

COLOUR
TIME

MUSIC

THE GADGETS AND TECH WE WANTED

Beeper
Car phone
Cordless phone
Discman
Game Boy
Hitclip
Imac

Laserjet printer
Minidisc
Nano pet
Nintendo
Nokia phone
Pager
Palm pilot

PlayStation
Speak and Spell
Talkboy
Walkman
Yak Bak

R	E	T	N	I	R	P	T	E	J	R	E	S	A	L
A	S	O	H	Y	O	B	K	L	A	T	C	A	M	I
E	C	A	R	P	H	O	N	E	O	E	K	C	L	L
N	I	G	N	Y	N	N	D	N	L	S	O	I	L	O
E	O	N	A	H	A	I	A	W	A	R	K	A	E	A
T	P	K	I	N	S	K	A	N	D	L	C	M	P	A
G	O	P	I	C	R	L	B	L	O	S	M	P	S	M
A	S	L	M	A	K	E	E	A	I	P	I	T	D	N
M	A	A	I	M	P	S	P	D	K	L	E	A	N	I
E	N	S	A	P	S	H	I	E	C	E	D	T	A	N
B	K	N	T	P	M	N	O	T	E	E	N	I	K	T
O	A	I	H	O	I	L	I	N	K	B	S	P	A	E
Y	E	O	S	M	N	H	A	P	E	R	S	M	E	N
T	N	T	P	R	I	A	K	P	R	E	G	A	P	D
E	P	L	A	Y	S	T	A	T	I	O	N	S	S	O

Solution on page 127

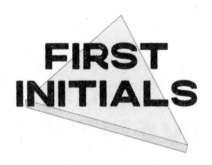

FIRST INITIALS

The Theme Songs
We Sung Along To

You definitely know the tunes but do you
know the song titles *and* can you identify
them by their first initials?

1 I'⬜ A⬜⬜⬜⬜⬜ H⬜⬜⬜

2 I D⬜⬜⬜ W⬜⬜⬜
T⬜ W⬜⬜⬜

3 E⬜⬜⬜⬜⬜⬜⬜⬜⬜
Y⬜⬜ L⬜⬜⬜

4 I'⬜⬜ B⬜ T⬜⬜⬜⬜
F⬜⬜ Y⬜⬜

5 I⬚ T⬚⬚ S⬚⬚⬚⬚⬚

6 T⬚⬚ F⬚⬚⬚⬚
P⬚⬚⬚⬚⬚ O⬚
B⬚⬚-A⬚⬚

7 H⬚⬚ S⬚⬚⬚ I⬚
N⬚⬚ ?

8 T⬚⬚⬚⬚⬚
S⬚⬚⬚⬚⬚ A⬚⬚
S⬚⬚⬚⬚⬚⬚⬚
E⬚⬚⬚

Answers on page 120

CHARACTERS IN FRIENDS

Alice	Gunther	Pete
Chandler	Janice	Phoebe
Charlie	Joey	Rachel
David	Joshua	Richard
Emily	Kathy	Ross
Emma	Monica	Ursula
Frank Jr	Mr Heckles	

U	S	R	P	K	J	H	P	Y	H	T	A	K	E	U
S	R	M	D	D	R	E	E	C	L	E	H	C	A	R
D	R	A	H	C	I	R	T	L	O	H	H	E	M	J
O	Y	A	R	A	M	M	E	C	U	D	E	R	O	D
E	R	E	H	T	N	U	G	A	L	L	H	E	H	I
C	H	A	N	D	L	E	R	A	L	E	Y	N	R	N
A	H	E	H	A	M	R	H	M	C	I	S	U	C	E
H	C	B	T	I	E	I	E	K	D	C	C	H	Y	E
S	M	I	L	V	R	A	L	R	A	N	A	E	E	E
S	O	Y	R	M	A	E	H	J	J	R	D	C	I	E
N	N	D	R	F	S	L	O	E	L	K	I	L	B	A
O	I	R	O	R	A	S	U	I	K	N	N	E	A	E
R	C	A	S	M	H	C	E	S	A	J	O	A	I	C
L	A	E	S	U	R	Y	S	J	R	H	Y	Y	R	C
D	I	V	A	D	R	Y	H	E	P	U	C	C	A	F

Solution on page 127

CROSSWORD 15

Solve the clues and discover the
1990s anagram in the shaded boxes!

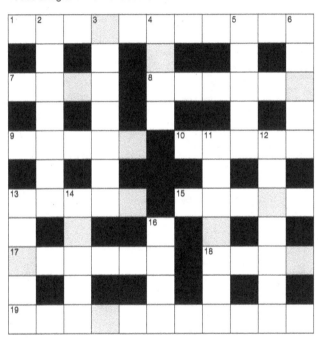

Across
1 Indicative (11)
7 Large edible fish (4)
8 Very drunk (slang) (6)
9 Lit-up (5)
10 Fisherman's bait? (5)
13 Male duck (5)
15 Extend a subscription (5)
17 Not quite (6)
18 Small crawling insects (4)
19 Irrational water fear (11)

Down
2 Junior (7)
3 Show-off (7)
4 Globes (4)
5 Private educator (5)
6 Lumps of earth (5)
11 Aromatic culinary herb (7)
12 Famous conductors (7)
13 Demise (5)
14 Equipped (5)
16 Red light instruction (4)

Solution on page 135

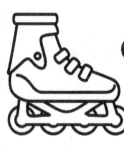
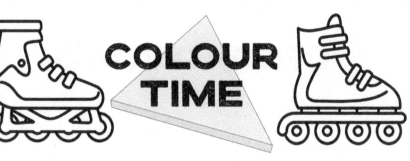
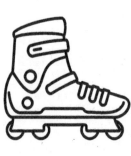

COLOUR TIME

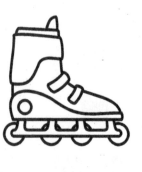
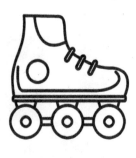
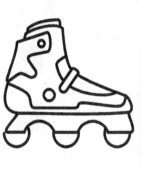

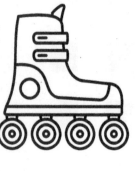
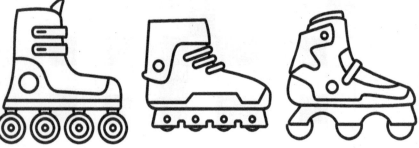
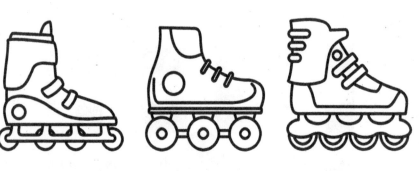

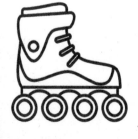
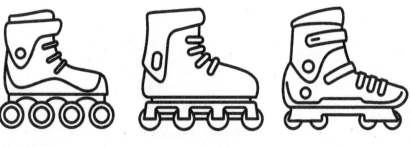

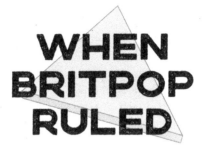

WHEN BRITPOP RULED

Anglocentric
Big Four
Blur
Boo Radleys
Cast
Catatonia
Cool Britannia

Cornershop
Definitely Maybe
Elastica
Guitar
James
Lush
Oasis

Parklife
Pulp
Rivalry
Rock
Suede
Union Jack

R	T	D	A	C	I	T	S	A	L	E	G	R	A	N
C	I	R	T	N	E	C	O	L	G	N	A	C	U	C
K	O	T	A	N	O	A	S	I	S	K	B	C	O	L
P	O	H	S	R	E	N	R	O	C	O	R	O	A	A
S	A	G	B	L	U	R	C	L	O	C	L	A	O	I
C	P	I	U	L	L	K	B	R	R	B	I	T	C	N
A	A	S	E	I	C	N	A	I	R	O	B	L	L	O
P	R	F	S	O	T	D	V	I	S	I	T	L	O	T
U	K	C	R	O	L	A	T	C	T	O	S	U	I	A
L	L	K	R	E	L	A	R	A	L	U	A	S	M	T
P	I	D	Y	R	N	J	A	M	E	S	C	H	O	A
A	F	S	Y	N	U	N	I	O	N	J	A	C	K	C
D	E	F	I	N	I	T	E	L	Y	M	A	Y	B	E
A	R	A	D	Y	S	U	E	D	E	S	M	S	E	I
U	S	L	E	C	B	I	G	F	O	U	R	C	O	K

Solution on page 128

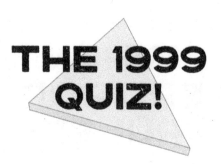

THE 1999 QUIZ!

1 Sunnydale High featured in which TV show?

2 Which video game console was selling the most at the end of the 1990s?

3 In *Dawson's Creek*, Joey and Pacey finally declare their love for each other and decided to spend the summer on Pacey's yacht. What is the name of his boat?

4 What was the name of the bestselling Backstreet Boys' single released in 1999?

5 Which band released 'Supernatural', featuring collaborations with CeeLo Green and Eric Clapton, among others?

6 Which 1999 movie premiered at the Sundance Film Festival listing some actors as either 'missing' or 'deceased'?

7 Can you remember all nine of the girls' names sung in Lou Begas' 1999 hit 'Mambo No. 5'?

8 Who reminded us to wear sunscreen?

9 Which *Simpsons* character was killed off because of a pay raise dispute with the voice actress, Maggie Roswell?

10 Who posed in her underwear with a purple Teletubby for the cover of *Rolling Stone* magazine?

Answers on page 118

A TRIP TO BLOCKBUSTER VIDEO

Blue and yellow	Fine	Rewind
Browse	Ice cream	Shelf
Candy	Membership card	Snack
Carpet	New release	Trailer
Cartoon	Popcorn	Two weeks
Cassette	Rental	Video
Disc	Return	

```
R E T U R N E T Y O C S D C E
C A S S E T T E E C N A V S E
N W K F I N E D E A T E N I E
E S W O R B I S C D F U O D R
R L S P S V N K K N V L W R Y
D R A C P I H S R E B M E M D
C A R P E T S U H W E N L H I
H P O P C O R N S L T W R U S
N R E L I A R T R A R B O L I
O A T W I K L E L H E U S W H
O S I S R I C E C R E A M E T
T E S A E L E R W E N I N R D
R W O L L E Y D N A E U L B C
A E I T S T E R E W I N D B M
C D E P O R A V C C I E O E E
```

Solution on page 128

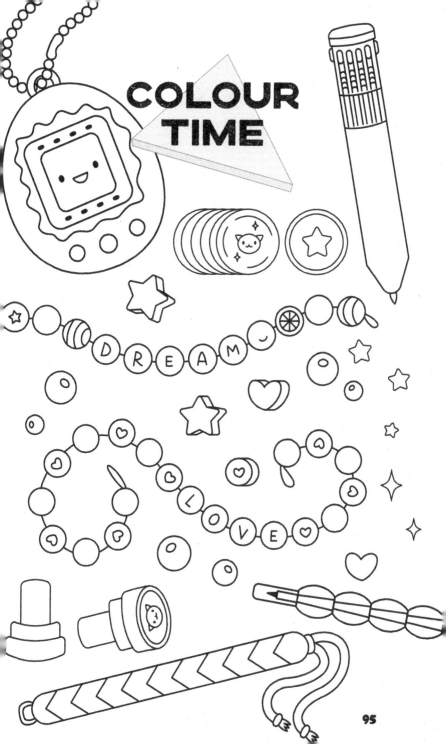

COLOUR
TIME

DREAM

LOVE

95

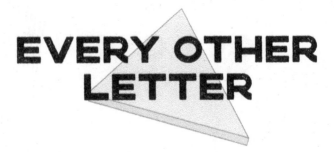

EVERY OTHER LETTER

Jim Carrey Movies

He was the crazy-faced comic icon of the 1990s.
Restore the names of these Jim Carrey movies
by placing a letter into each gap.

1 A ☐ E ☐ E ☐ T ☐ R ☐ :
☐ E ☐ D ☐ T ☐ C ☐ I ☐ E

2 ☐ H ☐ M ☐ S ☐

3 ☐ U ☐ B ☐ N ☐
D ☐ M ☐ E ☐

4 B ☐ T ☐ A ☐
F ☐ R ☐ V ☐ R

5 T ⬚ E ⬚ A L ⬚ G ⬚ Y

6 ⬚ I ⬚ R ⬚ I ⬚ R

7 T ⬚ E T ⬚ U ⬚ A ⬚
   S ⬚ O ⬚

8 S ⬚ M ⬚ N ⬚ I ⬚ C ⬚

9 ⬚ A ⬚ O ⬚ T ⬚ E
   ⬚ O ⬚ N

Answers on page 120

THE TOYS WE MOST WANTED

Beanie Babies
Big Yellow Teapot
Bop It
Dream Phone
Furbies
Gameboy

Glo Worm
Micro Machines
Mouse Trap
Mr Frosty
My Little Pony
Nintendo

Pogs
Polly Pocket
Tamagotchi
Trolls

B	P	I	G	A	O	S	M	O	U	S	E	T	R	A	P	M
E	D	O	C	D	O	T	O	M	R	O	W	O	L	G	S	L
A	T	U	M	N	Y	A	E	A	M	T	B	P	R	M	E	R
N	D	O	L	O	O	M	L	I	L	T	T	G	Y	O	N	S
I	R	U	P	N	Y	A	B	B	L	E	E	O	I	L	I	I
E	E	Y	I	A	S	G	T	O	F	K	C	N	Y	I	H	Y
B	A	T	M	N	E	O	Y	P	M	C	M	N	O	A	C	S
A	M	S	T	O	M	T	N	I	R	O	O	E	D	S	A	I
B	P	O	G	R	B	C	W	T	C	P	M	T	N	E	M	O
I	H	R	Y	A	O	H	L	O	E	Y	G	O	E	I	O	W
E	O	F	I	G	M	I	E	L	L	L	E	R	T	B	R	E
S	N	R	G	B	M	E	T	R	O	L	L	S	N	R	C	D
O	E	M	M	M	R	T	B	A	S	O	E	T	I	U	I	W
I	T	G	P	Y	I	H	I	O	I	P	R	Y	N	F	M	Y
P	N	O	O	L	R	O	I	R	Y	L	M	G	G	P	F	B
C	P	T	Y	I	T	P	O	G	S	O	A	O	R	I	B	O
I	I	M	C	G	M	M	H	D	R	E	Y	M	O	N	B	O

Solution on page 128

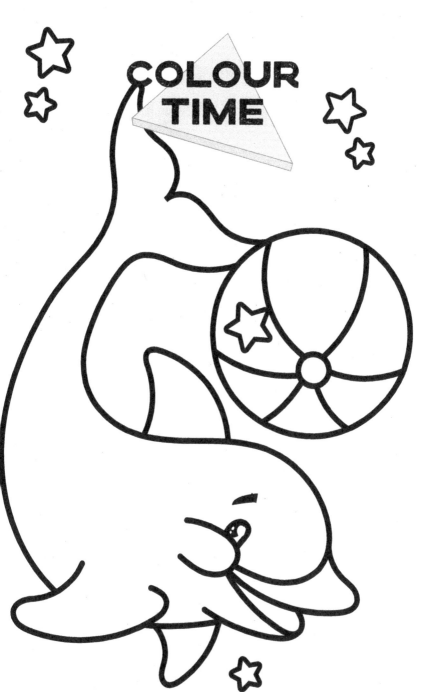

COLOUR TIME

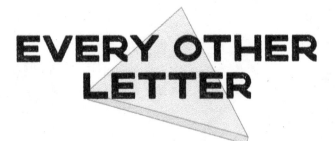

EVERY OTHER LETTER

Cult Indie Films

Can you fill in the missing letters to reveal the movies we felt cool for watching?

1 D ☐ Z ☐ D ☐ N ☐
C ☐ N ☐ U ☐ E ☐

2 R ☐ A ☐ I ☐ Y ☐ I ☐ E ☐

3 E ☐ P ☐ R ☐
R ☐ C ☐ R ☐ S

4 H ☐ C ☐ E ☐ S

5 M ☐ O ☐ N ☐ R ☐ V ☐ T ☐
I ☐ A ☐ O

6 T ☐ U ☐ R ☐ M ☐ N ☐ E

7 W ☐ A ☐ 'S ☐ A ☐ I ☐ G
☐ I ☐ B ☐ R ☐ G ☐ A ☐ E

8 T ☐ E ☐ ☐ I ☐
☐ L ☐ B ☐ W ☐ K ☐

9 G ☐ O ☐ W ☐ L ☐
H ☐ N ☐ I ☐ G

10 S ☐ A ☐ L ☐ W
☐ R ☐ V ☐

Answers on page 120

DISNEY OF THE 1990s

A Bug's Life
Aladdin
Blank Check
Cool Runnings
Darkwing Duck

Flubber
Hercules
Hocus Pocus
Mighty Ducks
Mulan

Pocahontas
Talespin
Tarzan
The Lion King
Toy Story

A	K	C	E	H	C	K	N	A	L	B	L	H	S	P	H	B
Y	R	S	P	C	L	H	O	C	U	S	P	O	C	U	S	E
U	S	T	A	P	O	K	A	G	I	F	L	U	B	B	E	R
S	G	O	N	T	D	E	U	L	K	R	I	B	A	R	N	G
E	N	T	K	P	N	A	Y	U	R	T	S	P	A	O	M	L
L	I	A	A	S	L	O	R	N	N	H	K	S	P	L	G	E
U	N	R	B	L	Y	R	H	K	Y	E	D	U	P	H	C	N
C	N	Z	U	C	E	O	N	A	W	L	C	L	S	N	B	I
R	U	A	G	E	N	S	Y	U	C	I	T	M	I	U	U	D
E	R	N	S	O	S	M	P	L	G	O	N	C	O	U	B	D
H	L	L	L	S	N	B	M	I	P	N	P	G	S	K	B	A
E	O	L	I	U	D	U	K	U	N	K	I	P	D	T	K	L
D	O	W	F	O	L	D	L	O	R	I	S	R	A	U	B	A
R	C	R	E	A	U	K	Y	P	G	N	U	N	E	N	C	N
K	C	C	N	O	A	P	Y	U	C	G	O	T	O	R	C	K
F	I	B	P	M	I	G	H	T	Y	D	U	C	K	S	E	S
L	A	Y	R	O	T	S	Y	O	T	Y	Y	T	B	G	I	R

Solution on page 129

LOCATIONS IN FRIENDS

Atlantic City
Barbados
Bermuda
Bloomingdales
Central Park

Las Vegas
London
Long Island
Montauk
Moondance Diner

Newark Airport
Ohio
Plaza Hotel
Tulsa
Vermont

D	C	O	H	K	O	I	A	A	O	N	A	C	T	M
S	S	A	G	E	V	S	A	L	A	A	D	E	R	O
K	E	P	D	V	N	O	C	D	E	G	C	N	O	O
U	A	L	W	N	U	L	U	S	V	E	A	T	P	N
N	T	A	A	M	A	M	O	M	T	A	N	R	R	D
A	L	Z	M	D	R	L	L	H	N	T	A	A	I	A
E	A	A	K	E	G	N	S	O	E	S	P	L	A	N
M	N	H	B	A	O	N	D	I	O	D	R	P	K	C
O	T	O	T	L	S	N	I	D	G	S	N	A	R	E
N	I	T	P	N	O	L	A	M	H	N	L	R	A	D
T	C	E	A	L	O	B	U	L	O	I	O	K	W	I
A	C	L	N	C	R	M	G	T	N	O	O	L	E	N
U	I	E	S	A	W	A	R	D	L	I	L	R	N	E
K	T	M	B	A	D	I	M	E	H	A	R	B	T	R
O	Y	L	A	U	N	E	K	O	V	L	N	P	T	L

Solution on page 129

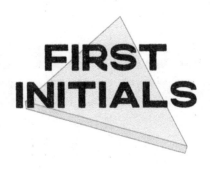

Romcoms

Can you work out which 1990s romcoms have been clued below, where only the initials of each film's title have been given? 'Jerry Maguire', for example, would be given as 'J M'.

1 F W A A F

_____

2 T T I H A Y

_____

3 T S A M

_____

4 H S G H G B

_____

5 R A M H S R

_____

6 M B F W

_____

7 W Y W S

_____

8 B I A C

_____

9 A G A I G

_____

10 N B K

_____

Answers on page 120

CROSSWORD 16

Solve the clues and discover the
1990s anagram in the shaded boxes!

Across
1 Device for boiling water (6)
4 Random-number cube (4)
6 Graduates (6)
7 Nigh (4)
8 Acid counterpart (6)
11 Tiny amount (4)
12 Cash register (4)
13 Go for the opponent's goal (6)
16 Manure (4)
17 Overlook (6)
18 Bawdy (4)
19 Required (6)

Down
1 Eucalyptus-eater (5)
2 Thickest part of a tree (5)
3 Abolition (11)
4 Tooth doctor (7)
5 Disordered (7)
9 Spare time (7)
10 Asserted (7)
14 Avert (5)
15 Pummel dough (5)

Solution on page 136

OUR FAVOURITE CARTOONS

Animaniacs
Captain Planet
Daria
Ducktales
Family Guy

Hey Arnold
Inspector Gadget
Johnny Bravo
Powerpuff Girls
Ren And Stimpy

Rugrats
South Park
The Simpsons

```
N S L R I G F F U P R E W O P T M
I Y P M I T S D N A N E R H O E O
U N O G S S Y A S N N O H E K N I
N S S V A C U E I L G E H Y S A D
R K U P A I A G A R I A K A M L U
U R R S E R I I C T A U P R O P C
G S A D T C B I N B M D A N F N K
R Y B N C L T Y O A A R B O U I T
A S K T G U E O N E M N I L E A A
T O O E R B E G R N Y I O D Y T L
S U R P P N E C Y G H P N Y Y P E
G T P H R E N A Y C A O Y A M A S
T H E S I M P S O N S D J I U C U
O P R H A A T E N A F T G E O N A
H A T Y U G Y L I M A F S E S R R
R R T A Y L A A K E N H H N T I T
R K N P Y I F L P N I K R L C A U
```

Solution on page 129

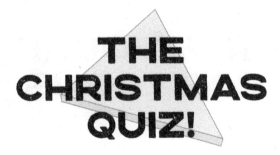

THE CHRISTMAS QUIZ!

1 Who played Howard Langston in the 1996 Christmas comedy *Jingle All the Way*?

2 Who released their 'Home for Christmas' album in 1998?

3 What did Destiny's Child get on the sixth day of Christmas according to their hit song, '8 Days of Christmas'?

4 In *Friends*, when he discovers that all of the Santa costumes have been rented out, what costume does Ross hire instead?

5 Which Christmas song, originally released in 1994, has surpassed 16 million total worldwide sales and was rereleased in 2010?

6 Which toy, that was a bestseller in December 1998, was later briefly banned by America's National Security Agency, apparently over concerns it could be a security threat?

7 How many days does it take Kevin's mother to get back home to him in the first *Home Alone* movie?

8 What was the biggest-selling toy of 1993 – also a prop featured in Christmas sequel *Home Alone 2*?

9 Which film, originally released in 1947, was remade and released for Christmas 1994, co-produced and written by John Hughes?

10 Which Muppet plays Charles Dickens in 1992's *The Muppet Christmas Carol*?

Answers on page 118

CROSSWORD

17

Solve the clues and discover the 1990s anagram in the shaded boxes!

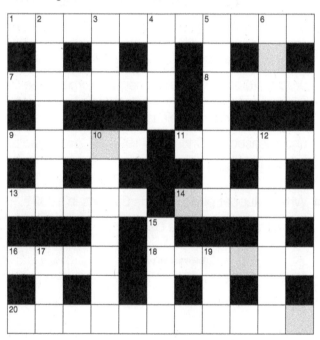

Across
1 Name (11)
7 Exaggerate (6)
8 Operator (4)
9 General idea (5)
11 Clock's hourly sound (5)
13 Wandering person (5)
14 Employing (5)
16 Type of gemstone (4)
18 Misgivings (6)
20 Yearly celebration (11)

Down
2 Destitution (7)
3 It's essential for listening (3)
4 Repeating program code (4)
5 Contacts (7)
6 Naturally occurring mineral aggregate (3)
10 Short spiral pasta (7)
12 Computer display (7)
15 Upper hand (4)
17 Small brooch (3)
19 Opposite of downs (3)

Solution on page 136

THE ERA OF THE SUPERMODEL

Cindy Crawford	Heidi Klum	Nadja Auermann
Claudia Schiffer	Karen Mulder	Naomi Campbell
Elle Macphearson	Kate Moss	Tyra Banks
Eva Herzigova	Kristen Mcmenamy	Yasmeen Ghauri

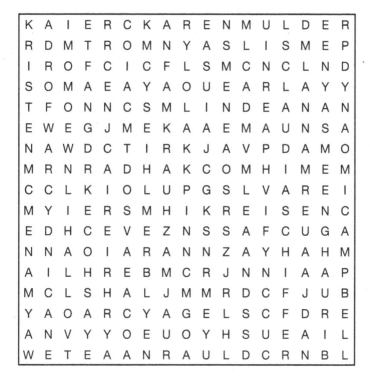

K	A	I	E	R	C	K	A	R	E	N	M	U	L	D	E	R
R	D	M	T	R	O	M	N	Y	A	S	L	I	S	M	E	P
I	R	O	F	C	I	C	F	L	S	M	C	N	C	L	N	D
S	O	M	A	E	A	Y	A	O	U	E	A	R	L	A	Y	Y
T	F	O	N	N	C	S	M	L	I	N	D	E	A	N	A	N
E	W	E	G	J	M	E	K	A	A	E	M	A	U	N	S	A
N	A	W	D	C	T	I	R	K	J	A	V	P	D	A	M	O
M	R	N	R	A	D	H	A	K	C	O	M	H	I	M	E	M
C	C	L	K	I	O	L	U	P	G	S	L	V	A	R	E	I
M	Y	I	E	R	S	M	H	I	K	R	E	I	S	E	N	C
E	D	H	C	E	V	E	Z	N	S	S	A	F	C	U	G	A
N	N	A	O	I	A	R	A	N	N	Z	A	Y	H	A	H	M
A	I	L	H	R	E	B	M	C	R	J	N	N	I	A	A	P
M	C	L	S	H	A	L	J	M	M	R	D	C	F	J	U	B
Y	A	O	A	R	C	Y	A	G	E	L	S	C	F	D	R	E
A	N	V	Y	Y	O	E	U	O	Y	H	S	U	E	A	I	L
W	E	T	E	A	A	N	R	A	U	L	D	C	R	N	B	L

Solution on page 130

COLOUR
TIME

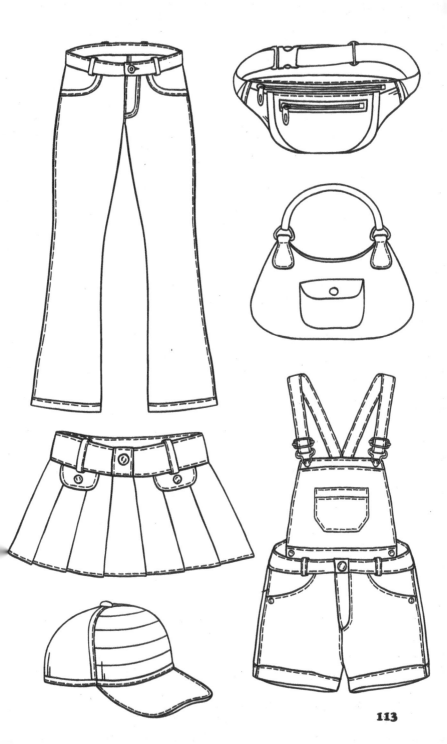

READY FOR THE ANSWERS?

The Quizzes

8. A Royale with cheese
9. Tia and Tamera
10. *Forrest Gump*

p.54 The 1995 Quiz!

1. Oasis with 'Roll with It' and Blur with 'Country House'. Blur's song sold more copies.
2. Tommy Lee
3. Robbie Williams/ Take That
4. Tan
5. A 'Baldwin'
6. Match.com
7. The stuffed crust
8. O J Simpson
9. 'Gangsta's Paradise'
10. *Casper*

p.62 The 1996 Quiz!

1. 'Macarena'
2. *Romeo + Juliet*
3. Seven
4. Lauryn Hill, Pras Michel and Wyclef Jean
5. Shave her head
6. Dolly the sheep
7. Ask Jeeves
8. *Space Jam*
9. *The Craft*
10. Madonna

p.66 The Song Lyrics Quiz!

1. Lauryn Hill ('Ready or Not' – The Fugees)

2. Courtney Love ('Celebrity Skin' – Hole)
3. Skee-Lo ('I Wish')
4. The Backstreet Boys ('I Want It That Way')
5. Whigfield ('Saturday Night')
6. Alanis Morissette
7. Jarvis Cocker ('Year 2000' – Pulp)
8. Ibiza ('We're Going to Ibiza' – The Venga Boys)
9. Anthony Kiedis ('Under the Bridge' – The Red Hot Chili Peppers)
10. Bryan Adams ('The Summer of '69')
11. Brandy and Monica ('The Boy Is Mine')
12. Liam Gallagher ('Roll with It' – Oasis)

p.72 The 1997 quiz!

1. 'Torn'
2. Tamagotchi
3. 2007
4. Hanson
5. 'Everybody (Backstreet's Back)'
6. The Teletubbies (Dipsy, Laa-Laa, Tinky-Winky and Po)
7. *Men in Black*
8. LeAnn Rimes
9. Christopher 'The Notorious B.I.G.' Wallace
10. Ellen DeGeneres

The Letter Puzzles

4. *Grace* by Jeff Buckley
5. *Dookie* by Green Day
6. *The Slim Shady LP* by Eminem
7. *(What's the Story) Morning Glory?* by Oasis
8. *The Score* by Fugees
9. *Jagged Little Pill* by Alanis Morissette
10. *The Ghost of Tom Joad* by Bruce Springsteen

p.40 Missing Vowels:
The Most-Watched *X-Files*
Episodes

1. 'Leonard Betts'
2. 'Redux'
3. 'Detour'
4. 'Unusual Suspects'
5. 'Schizogeny'
6. 'Never Again'
7. 'The Rain King'
8. 'The Sixth Extinction'
9. 'Fresh Bones'
10. 'Small Potatoes'

p.50 Missing Vowels:
Sports Stars

1. Michael Jordan
2. Andre Agassi
3. Serena Williams
4. Shaquille O'Neal
5. Ronaldo
6. Brett Favre
7. Mia Hamm
8. Mike Tyson

9. Michelle Kwan
10. Eric Cantona

p.60 First Initials:
Horror Films

1. *I Know What You Did Last Summer*
2. *The Silence of the Lambs*
3. *The Blair Witch Project*
4. *The People Under the Stairs*
5. *The Hand That Rocks the Cradle*
6. *Interview with the Vampire*
7. *Wes Craven's New Nightmare*
8. *The Sixth Sense*
9. *Bram Stoker's Dracula*
10. *It*

p.76 Every Other Letter:
Comedians

1. Jim Carrey
2. Chris Rock
3. Dave Chapelle
4. Adam Sandler
5. Margaret Cho
6. Mike Myers
7. Jerry Seinfeld
8. Steve Harvey
9. Martin Lawrence
10. Joan Collins

p.86 First Initials:
The Theme Songs We Sang
Along To

1. 'I'm Always Here'
   (*Baywatch*)
2. 'I Don't Want to Wait'
   (*Dawson's Creek*)
3. 'Everywhere You Look'
   (*Full House*)
4. 'I'll Be There for You'
   (*Friends*)
5. 'In the Street' (*The '70s
   Show*)
6. 'The Fresh Prince of Bel-Air'
   (*The Fresh Prince of Bel-Air*)
7. 'How Soon Is Now?'
   (*Charmed*)
8. 'Tossed Salads and
   Scrambled Eggs' (*Frasier*)

p.96 Every Other Letter:
Jim Carrey Movies

1. *Ace Ventura: Pet Detective*
2. *The Mask*
3. *Dumb and Dumber*
4. *Batman Forever*
5. *The Cable Guy*
6. *Liar Liar*
7. *The Truman Show*
8. *Simon Birch*
9. *Man on the Moon*

p.100 Every Other Letter:
Cult Indie Films

1. *Dazed and Confused*
2. *Reality Bites*
3. *Empire Records*
4. *Hackers*
5. *My Own Private Idaho*
6. *True Romance*
7. *What's Eating Gilbert Grape*
8. *The Big Lebowski*
9. *Good Will Hunting*
10. *Shallow Grave*

p.104 First Initials:
Romcoms

1. *Four Weddings and a
   Funeral*
2. *Ten Things I Hate About
   You*
3. *There's Something About
   Mary*
4. *How Stella Got Her
   Groove Back*
5. *Romy and Michelle's High
   School Reunion*
6. *My Best Friend's Wedding*
7. *While You Were Sleeping*
8. *But I'm a Cheerleader*
9. *As Good As It Gets*
10. *Never Been Kissed*

The Wordsearches

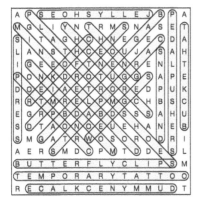

p.8
The Things We Wore

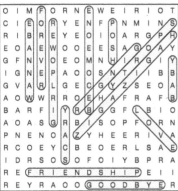

p.12
Girl Power

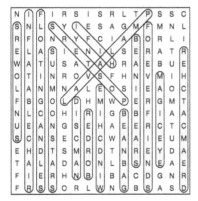

p.19
Our Bedroom Decor Essentials

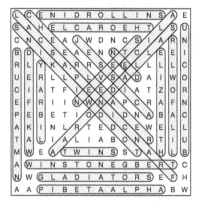

p.22
Sweet Valley High

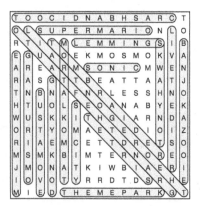

p.26
The Games We Got Addicted To

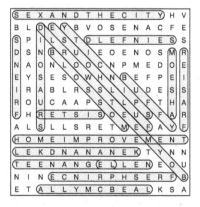

p.30
The Sitcoms We Watched Every Week

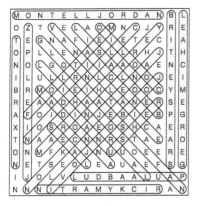

p.33
1990s Music Icons

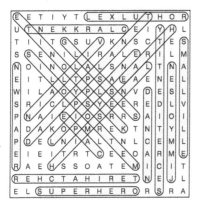

p.36
The New Adventures of Superman

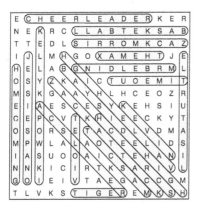

p.38
Saved by the Bell

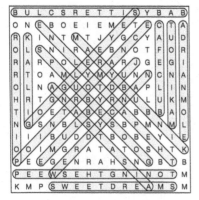

p.45
The Books We Loved as Teens

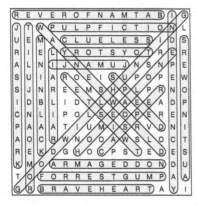

p.49
1990s Blockbuster Movies

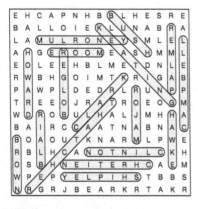

p.53
The PMs and Presidents of the 1990s

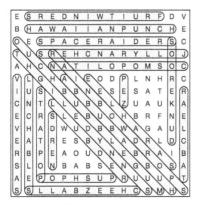

p.57
The Drinks and Snacks We Craved

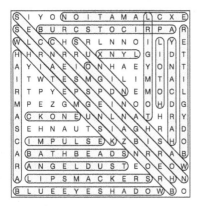

p.59
Our Beauty Must-Haves

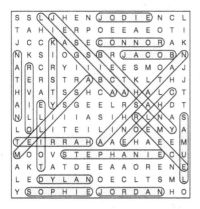

p.65
Popular Names in the 1990s

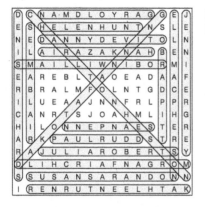

p.69
Friends Guest Stars

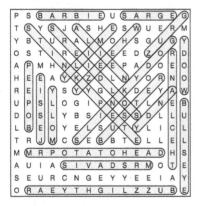

p.74
Toy Story 1 and 2

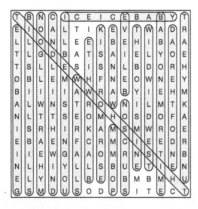

p.78
Floor Fillers of the 1990s

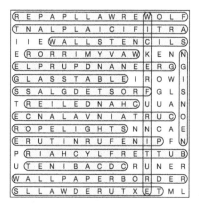

p.82
The Coolest 1990s Decor

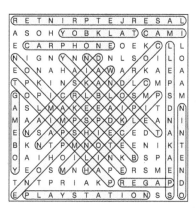

p.85
The Gadgets and Tech We Wanted

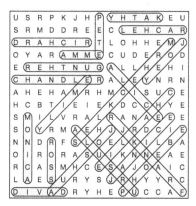

p.88
Characters in Friends

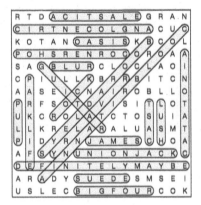

p.91
When Britpop Ruled

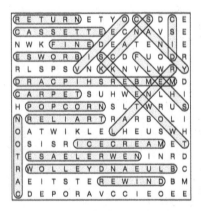

p.94
A Trip to Blockbuster Video

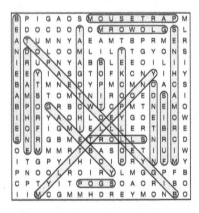

p.98
The Toys We Most Wanted

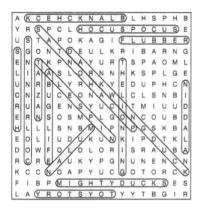

p.102
Disney of the 1990s

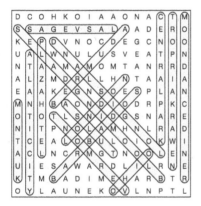

p.103
Locations in Friends

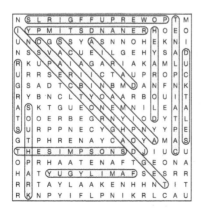

p.107
Our Favourite Cartoons

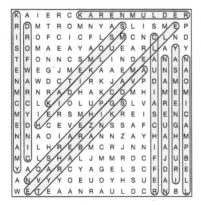

p.111
The Era of the
Supermodel

The Crosswords

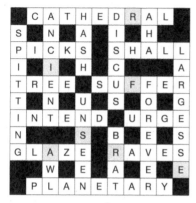

p.10
Crossword 1

Anagram:
FRASIER

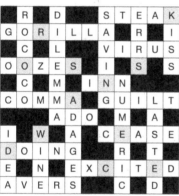

p.13
Crossword 2

Anagram:
DAWSON'S CREEK

p.18
Crossword 3

Anagram:
ALLY MCBEAL

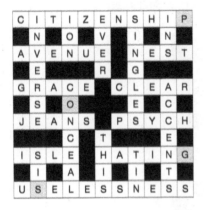

p.21
Crossword 4

Anagram:
POGS

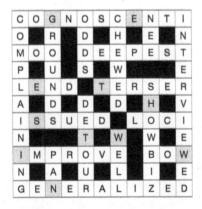

p.27
Crossword 5

Anagram:
FRIENDS

p.32
Crossword 6

Anagram:
THE WEST WING

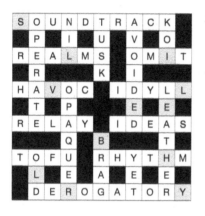

p.37
Crossword 7

Anagram:
BEVERLY HILLS

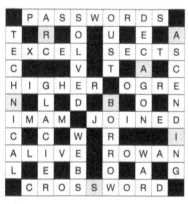

p.44
Crossword 8

Anagram:
SABRINA

p.52
Crossword 9

Anagram:
SEX AND THE CITY

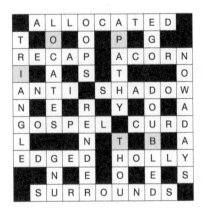

p.58
Crossword 10

Anagram:
BOP IT

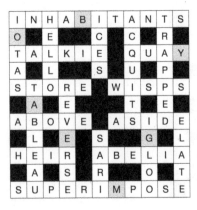

p.68
Crossword 11

Anagram:
GAMEBOY

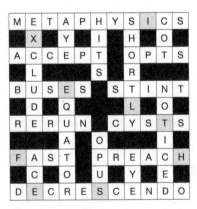

p.70
Crossword 12

Anagram:
THE X-FILES

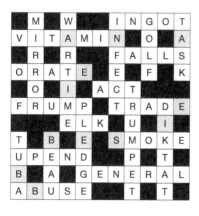

p.75
Crossword 13

Anagram:
BEANIE BABIES

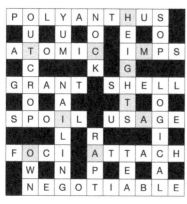

p.83
Crossword 14

Anagram:
TAMAGOTCHI

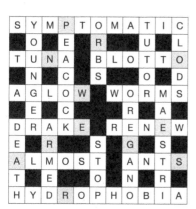

p.89
Crossword 15

Anagram:
POWER RANGERS

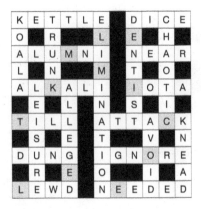

p.106
Crossword 16

Anagram:

TICKLE ME ELMO

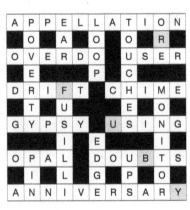

p.110
Crossword 17

Anagram:
FURBY

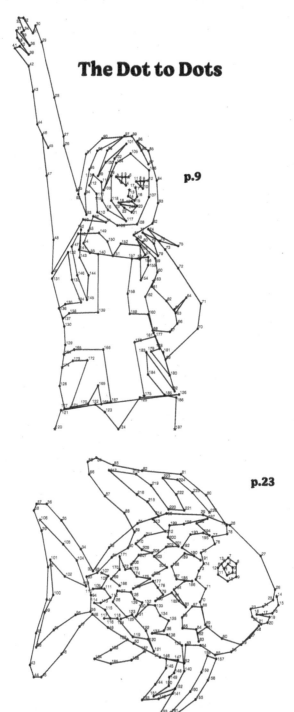

The Dot to Dots

p.9

p.23

137

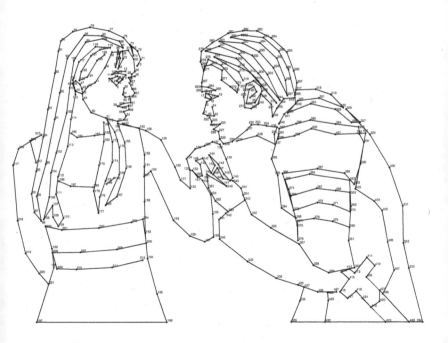

p.42

p.48

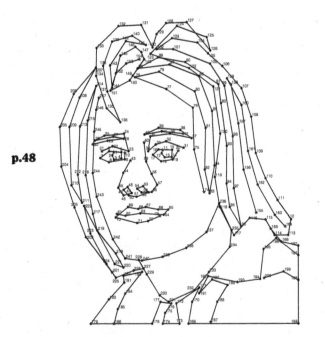

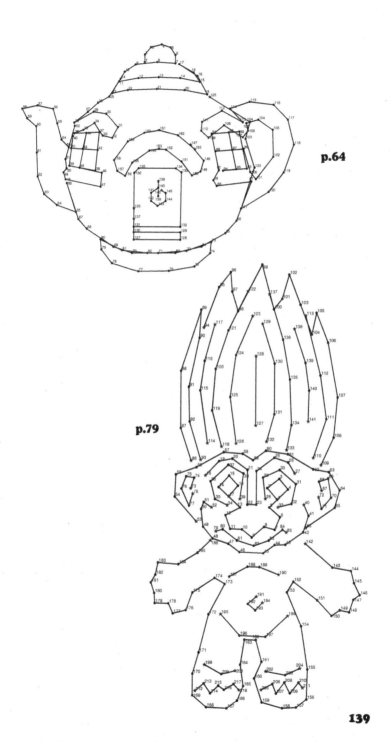

p.64

p.79

139

Published in 2023 by Pop Press,
an imprint of Ebury Publishing
20 Vauxhall Bridge Road
London SW1V 2SA

Pop Press is part of the Penguin Random House group of companies
whose addresses can be found at global.penguinrandomhouse.com

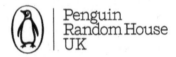

First published by Pop Press in 2023

www.penguin.co.uk

A CIP catalogue record for this book is available from the British Library

ISBN 9781529925517

Printed and bound in Great Britain by Clays Ltd, Elcograf S.p.A.

The authorised representative in the EEA is Penguin Random House Ireland,
Morrison Chambers, 32 Nassau Street, Dublin D02 YH68

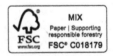

MIX
Paper | Supporting
responsible forestry
FSC® C018179

Penguin Random House is committed to a sustainable future
for our business, our readers and our planet. This book is
made from Forest Stewardship Council® certified paper.